HERBAL TINCTURES FOR BEGINNERS

A comprehensive handbook for making, using and benefiting from herbal extracts for well-being

TERESA MILLER

COPYRIGHT ©

All rights reserved.

No part of this book may be reproduced in any form or by any electronic or mechanical means, including information storage and retrieval systems, without permission in writing from the publisher, except by a reviewer who may quote brief passages in a review.

The information contained in this book is based on the author's research and experience. While the author has made every effort to provide accurate and up-to-date information, errors and omissions may occur. The author and publisher assume no responsibility for any errors or omissions or for any actions taken based on the information contained in this book.

The information contained in this book is provided "as is," without warranty of any kind, express or implied, including but not limited to the warranties of merchantability, fitness for a particular purpose, or non-infringement. In no event shall the author or publisher be liable for any claim, damages, or other liability, whether in an action of contract, tort, or otherwise, arising from, out of, or in connection with the book or the use or other dealings in the book.

TABLE OF CONTENTS

INTRODUCTION

In the realm of natural remedies and holistic wellness, herbal tinctures stand as age-old elixirs encapsulating the essence of botanical healing. For centuries, civilizations across the globe have harnessed the power of herbs, roots, and flowers, distilling their potent properties into concentrated liquid forms known as tinctures. These alchemical concoctions have traversed time, bridging the gap between traditional herbal wisdom and contemporary healthcare practices.

What exactly are herbal tinctures? At their core, they are concentrated herbal extracts, typically preserved in alcohol, glycerin, or vinegar. Through a meticulous process of maceration and extraction, these liquid essences capture the medicinal attributes of plants, offering a concentrated dose of their therapeutic benefits.

The significance of herbal tinctures transcends eras, weaving through the annals of history into our modern-day quest for holistic well-being. In traditional medicine systems like Ayurveda, Traditional Chinese Medicine (TCM), and Native American healing practices, tinctures have been revered as potent remedies, revered for their versatility and efficacy in addressing an array of health concerns.

In the tapestry of modern herbal medicine, tinctures hold a special place. They offer a convenient and efficient means of accessing the healing potential of herbs in a concentrated form. Unlike teas or capsules, tinctures present a more potent and easily absorbable format, enabling swift assimilation of herbal goodness into our bodies.

Furthermore, the adaptability of herbal tinctures caters to diverse needs – whether seeking relief from common ailments, enhancing overall vitality, or complementing conventional treatments. Their versatility allows for custom blends tailored to individual requirements, catering to a spectrum of physical, mental, and emotional imbalances.

The beauty of herbal tinctures lies in their adaptability. They can be tailored to suit individual needs, addressing an array of health concerns—from supporting immune health to promoting mental clarity and aiding in stress management. Their versatility and potency make them indispensable in holistic health practices, complementing modern treatments and empowering individuals on their wellness journeys.

As our collective consciousness embraces a return to nature's bounty and seeks alternatives to synthetic remedies, herbal tinctures emerge as beacons of natural wellness. Their resurgence in popularity echoes the innate human desire for connection with the Earth's gifts and the pursuit of a harmonious, balanced existence.

In this comprehensive guide, we embark on an exploration of herbal tinctures, delving into their creation, benefits, applications, and the timeless wisdom they encapsulate. Join us on this journey as we unlock the secrets of these botanical elixirs, offering pathways to healing, rejuvenation, and a deeper communion with nature's healing embrace.

CHAPTER ONE

WHAT ARE HERBAL TINCTURES?

Herbal tinctures are concentrated liquid extracts derived from herbs, plants, flowers, roots, or berries. These extracts are made by soaking the botanical material in a solvent, typically alcohol, glycerin, or vinegar, over a period of time to extract and preserve the active compounds and medicinal properties present in the plant material.

The tincturing process involves macerating or steeping the herbs in the chosen liquid solvent, allowing the active constituents—such as essential oils, alkaloids, flavonoids, and other beneficial compounds—to infuse into the solvent. This extraction process results in a highly concentrated liquid that retains the therapeutic properties of the herbs.

Once the extraction is complete, the liquid is usually strained to remove the solid plant material, leaving behind a potent herbal extract. Herbal tinctures are often stored in dark-colored glass bottles to protect them from light, which can degrade the active constituents, and are typically labeled with information regarding the herb used, the type of solvent, and the extraction ratio.

These tinctures are revered for their versatility, as they can be administered orally, added to beverages, used topically, or even incorporated into culinary preparations. They offer a convenient and efficient way to access the medicinal benefits of herbs, allowing for easy dosing and absorption, and are widely used in traditional and modern herbal medicine practices to support health and well-being.

SIGNIFICANCE OF HERBAL TINCTURES IN TRADITIONAL AND MODERN HERBAL MEDICINE

The significance of herbal tinctures in both traditional and modern herbal medicine is substantial, owing to their versatility, potency, and practicality in delivering the therapeutic properties of herbs. Here's an overview of their importance in both contexts:

Traditional Herbal Medicine:

• Historical Heritage: Herbal tinctures have deep roots in traditional healing systems worldwide. They've been used for centuries in diverse cultures such as Ayurveda, Traditional

Chinese Medicine (TCM), Native American healing practices, and European herbalism.

• Potency and Concentration: Tinctures are valued for their ability to concentrate the medicinal qualities of herbs. This potency allows for more effective treatment, requiring smaller doses compared to other herbal preparations like teas or decoctions.

• Long Shelf Life: Alcohol-based tinctures act as preservatives, extending the shelf life of herbs and allowing them to retain their potency for an extended period, making them an ideal choice for storage.

• Versatility and Customization: Herbalists often blend tinctures to create personalized remedies tailored to specific individual needs. The adaptability and combinatory nature of tinctures enable practitioners to address a wide range of health issues.

• Rapid Absorption: Tinctures are easily absorbed by the body, making their therapeutic effects quicker compared to other forms of herbal remedies. This faster absorption contributes to their effectiveness in providing relief for various ailments.

• Accessibility and Convenience: In contemporary herbal medicine, tinctures offer an accessible and user-friendly format for administering herbal remedies. They provide a straightforward method of consumption, allowing for easy integration into modern lifestyles.

• Precise Dosage and Administration: Tinctures enable precise dosing, making it easier for individuals to regulate and adjust their intake according to specific health needs, enhancing safety and effectiveness.

• Supportive Complement to Modern Medicine: Herbal tinctures are increasingly recognized as complementary to conventional medical treatments. They offer a natural alternative and can sometimes be used in tandem with pharmaceuticals to enhance overall wellness.

• Research and Validation: Ongoing scientific research continues to explore the efficacy and benefits of herbal tinctures. This modern scrutiny and validation of traditional knowledge contribute to their acceptance and integration into contemporary healthcare practices.

• Interest in Natural Remedies: As the interest in natural and holistic wellness grows, herbal tinctures gain prominence for their perceived effectiveness and minimal side effects compared to some synthetic medicines, aligning with the preferences of individuals seeking natural healing modalities.

The significance of herbal tinctures in both traditional and modern herbal medicine lies in their ability to harness the healing potential of plants, offering a bridge between ancient wisdom and current healthcare paradigms. Their adaptability, potency, and accessibility make them enduring allies in the pursuit of holistic well-being.

THE BENEFITS OF USING TINCTURES OVER OTHER HERBAL PREPARATIONS

Using tinctures offers several advantages over other herbal preparations, making them a preferred choice for many individuals seeking natural remedies. Here are the key benefits of using tinctures compared to other herbal forms:

• Concentration and Potency: Tinctures are highly concentrated extracts, containing a higher concentration of active compounds from herbs compared to other forms like teas or capsules. This concentration allows for more potent and effective doses, requiring smaller quantities for therapeutic effects.

• Rapid Absorption: Tinctures are easily absorbed by the body due to their liquid form. When taken orally, the active constituents are readily assimilated into the bloodstream, providing quicker therapeutic benefits compared to other herbal forms that need digestion or steeping time.

• Longer Shelf Life: Alcohol-based tinctures act as natural preservatives, extending the shelf life of herbs and maintaining their potency for an extended duration. Properly stored tinctures can last for several years, unlike some other herbal preparations that might lose potency relatively quickly.

• Convenient and Portable: Tinctures are convenient to use and easy to carry, making them practical for individuals with busy lifestyles. Their small, compact bottles can be transported easily, allowing for on-the-go access to herbal remedies.

• Precise Dosage Control: Tinctures enable precise dosage control, facilitating accurate administration of herbal extracts.

This control is especially beneficial when addressing specific health concerns or adjusting dosages according to individual needs.

• Versatility in Administration: Tinctures offer multiple administration methods. They can be taken directly under the tongue (sublingually), added to beverages, or even used topically, providing versatile applications for addressing various health issues.

• Customization and Blending: Herbalists often blend tinctures to create personalized formulations tailored to individual needs. This flexibility allows for the combination of different herbs to address specific health conditions, enhancing their efficacy.

• Quick Onset of Effects: Due to their rapid absorption, tinctures often provide quicker relief for acute conditions or symptoms, making them particularly useful for addressing immediate health concerns.

• Potential for Longer Extraction Times: Compared to teas or infusions, tinctures allow for longer extraction times, enabling a more comprehensive extraction of a broader range of active compounds from herbs, potentially enhancing their therapeutic effects.

These benefits collectively contribute to the popularity and effectiveness of tinctures as a preferred herbal remedy for various health issues, offering a potent, convenient, and customizable way to harness the healing properties of herbs.

A HISTORICAL OVERVIEW OF TINCTURES

The history of tinctures spans civilizations, cultures, and centuries, showcasing their enduring significance in herbal medicine and human healing practices. Here's an overview of the historical evolution of tinctures:

Ancient Origins:

• Ancient Civilizations: The use of herbal extracts and tinctures dates back to ancient civilizations such as Mesopotamia, Egypt, and China. These cultures documented the extraction of medicinal compounds from plants, often using alcohol or vinegar as solvents.

• Alchemical Practices: Alchemists in the Middle Ages played a crucial role in refining tincture-making methods. Their experimentation with herbal extractions and distillation techniques laid the groundwork for more sophisticated tincture preparations.

Traditional Herbal Medicine:

• Ayurveda: In ancient India, Ayurvedic texts dating back thousands of years detailed the preparation of herbal extracts, including tinctures, known as "rasa" or essences. These extracts were used to balance the body's doshas and treat various ailments.

• Traditional Chinese Medicine (TCM): TCM utilized herbal extracts, including tinctures, as part of its pharmacopeia. Herbalists prepared concentrated extracts to restore balance and treat illnesses, incorporating tinctures into formulations like herbal formulas and tonics.

• European Herbalism: Medieval European herbalists refined the art of tincture-making, documenting herbal preparations in texts like "The Herbal" by John Gerard and "The Complete Herbal" by Nicholas Culpeper. Tinctures gained popularity for their long shelf life and potent medicinal properties.

• Renaissance Alchemy: During the Renaissance, alchemical traditions continued to influence herbal medicine. Alchemists refined tincture-making techniques, aiming to extract the most potent medicinal essences from plants.

• Scientific Advancements: With the advancement of scientific understanding in the 19th and 20th centuries, herbal medicine faced challenges but continued to persist. Tinctures remained a part of herbalists' repertoire, adapting to changing medical practices.

Contemporary Resurgence:

• Revival of Herbalism: In recent decades, there has been a resurgence of interest in natural remedies and holistic health. This resurgence has led to a renewed appreciation for herbal tinctures, with herbalists, naturopaths, and individuals embracing these traditional remedies.

• Scientific Validation: Ongoing scientific research continues to explore the medicinal properties of herbs and their extracts, including tinctures. This modern scrutiny validates some of the historical claims about the efficacy of herbal tinctures, contributing to their acceptance in contemporary healthcare practices.

Throughout history, tinctures have endured as a testament to the healing potential of plants. Their evolution from ancient remedies to modern herbal medicine reflects a timeless tradition of harnessing nature's bounty for health and well-being, bridging ancient wisdom with contemporary healthcare practices.

THE TRADITIONAL USE OF HERBAL TINCTURES IN DIFFERENT CULTURES

Herbal tinctures have played a significant role in traditional medicine across various cultures, each with its unique practices and approaches to herbal healing. Here's a glimpse of their traditional use in different cultures:

Ayurveda (India):

• Rasa Shastra: Ayurveda, an ancient system of medicine in India, utilizes herbal tinctures known as "rasa" or "avaleha." These are concentrated liquid extracts made by macerating herbs in alcohol or other liquids. Rasa preparations are believed to contain the essence of plants and are used to balance doshas (body energies) and treat various ailments.

Traditional Chinese Medicine (TCM):

• Medicinal Formulas: TCM employs herbal tinctures, referred to as concentrated extracts or "fluid extracts," as components of complex medicinal formulas. These tinctures are derived from herbs soaked in alcohol or water and are administered in precise dosages to address specific health imbalances.

Native American Healing Practices:

• Medicinal Infusions: Native American healers prepared herbal tinctures and extracts by steeping various plants, roots, and barks in water or alcohol to create infusions. These tinctures were used ceremonially and medicinally, treating ailments ranging from digestive issues to respiratory problems and spiritual well-being.

European Herbalism:

• Alcohol-Based Extracts: Traditional European herbalists, particularly during the Middle Ages, developed tincture-making techniques using alcohol as a solvent. They recognized the preservative properties of alcohol and created concentrated herbal extracts, preserving the medicinal properties of herbs for extended periods.

African Herbal Medicine:

• Medicinal Brews: African traditional healers brewed tinctures or infusions using local plants and herbs, infusing them in water, alcohol, or other liquids. These preparations were used for treating various conditions, from infections to spiritual healing, often passed down through generations orally or through cultural practices.

South American Herbal Traditions:

• Amazonian Remedies: Indigenous cultures in the Amazon rainforest used tinctures prepared from rainforest plants and herbs. These tinctures were often consumed or applied topically and held spiritual and healing significance, aiding in treating specific illnesses and maintaining overall well-being.

In each of these cultures, herbal tinctures were employed as potent remedies, often integrated into complex medicinal formulations or administered individually. These traditional practices showcase the diverse methods of preparing and using herbal tinctures, highlighting their role in maintaining health and addressing a wide range of physical, emotional, and spiritual ailments within different cultural contexts.

COMMON HERBS USED IN TINCTURE MAKING

There is a wide array of herbs commonly used in tincture-making, each possessing unique medicinal properties and benefits. Here's an introduction to some commonly used herbs in tincture preparations:

1. Echinacea (Echinacea purpurea):

• Immune Support: Echinacea is renowned for its immune-boosting properties, often used to support the body's defense mechanisms against infections, colds, and flu.

2. Chamomile (Matricaria chamomilla):

• Calming and Digestive Aid: Chamomile tinctures are prized for their calming effects, aiding in relaxation, promoting sleep, and soothing digestive discomfort.

3. St. John's Wort (Hypericum perforatum):

• Mood Support: St. John's Wort tinctures are valued for their potential in supporting mood balance and alleviating mild depressive symptoms.

4. Peppermint (Mentha × piperita):

• Digestive Relief: Peppermint tinctures are known for their ability to ease digestive issues, including bloating, gas, and indigestion.

5. Valerian (Valeriana officinalis):

• Sleep Aid: Valerian root tinctures are used as natural sleep aids, assisting in promoting relaxation and improving sleep quality.

6. Ginger (Zingiber officinale):

• Digestive Health: Ginger tinctures are renowned for their digestive benefits, helping with nausea, motion sickness, and overall digestive comfort.

7. Milk Thistle (Silybum marianum):

• Liver Support: Milk Thistle tinctures are used to support liver health and aid in detoxification processes within the body.

8. Lemon Balm (Melissa officinalis):

• Stress Relief: Lemon Balm tinctures are known for their calming effects, often used to reduce stress, anxiety, and promote relaxation.

9. Elderberry (Sambucus nigra):

• Immune Enhancement: Elderberry tinctures are popular for their immune-boosting properties, particularly during cold and flu seasons.

10. Arnica (Arnica montana):

• Topical Relief: Arnica tinctures are primarily used topically to alleviate muscle soreness, bruises, and inflammation.

11. Turmeric (Curcuma longa):

• Anti-Inflammatory: Turmeric tinctures contain curcumin, known for their potent anti-inflammatory and antioxidant properties.

12. Hawthorn (Crataegus species):

• Heart Health: Hawthorn tinctures are recognized for supporting cardiovascular health and promoting a healthy heart.

These herbs represent just a fraction of the diverse range of plants and botanicals used in tincture-making. Each herb offers specific medicinal properties and can be combined or used individually to create herbal tinctures tailored to address various health concerns and promote overall well-being.

THE HERBS LISTED ABOVE BASED ON THEIR PROPERTIES

Here's a categorization of the herbs mentioned based on their primary properties and typical uses:

Immune Support:

- Echinacea

- Elderberry

Digestive Health:

- Chamomile

- Peppermint

- Ginger

Relaxation and Stress Relief:

- Chamomile

- St. John's Wort

- Lemon Balm

Sleep Aid:

• Valerian

Liver Support and Detoxification:

• Milk Thistle

Anti-Inflammatory and Pain Relief:

• Arnica

• Turmeric

Cardiovascular and Heart Health:

• Hawthorn

Each of these herbs exhibits distinct properties and health benefits, allowing herbalists and individuals interested in natural remedies to select and combine them in tincture preparations based on specific health needs or desired outcomes.

Different parts of plants, including leaves, flowers, roots, bark, and berries, contain unique concentrations of active compounds and medicinal properties. Each part can be utilized in tincture preparation, providing a diverse range of benefits. Here's a breakdown of how various plant parts are commonly used for tincture making:

Leaves and Flowers:

• Extraction Method: Leaves and flowers are often used fresh or dried for tincture-making. They contain essential oils, flavonoids, and other compounds that are easily extracted using alcohol or glycerin.

• Common Uses: Leaves and flowers are often utilized for their calming, aromatic, and antioxidant properties. Herbs like chamomile, lavender, and peppermint are frequently used in tinctures for relaxation, digestive support, or immune enhancement.

Roots:

• Extraction Method: Roots are generally tougher and contain more concentrated compounds, requiring a longer extraction period. They are often chopped, dried, and macerated for tincture preparation.

• Common Uses: Root tinctures, such as those made from ginger, valerian, or echinacea, are commonly used for digestive health, sleep aid, immune support, or anti-inflammatory purposes.

Bark:

• Extraction Method: Bark may contain potent compounds that require thorough extraction. It's often dried and ground before tincture preparation.

• Common Uses: Certain barks, like that from the slippery elm or cinnamon trees, may be used in tinctures for gastrointestinal health, soothing properties, or immune support.

• Extraction Method: Berries and fruit are usually macerated and soaked in alcohol or glycerin to extract their active constituents.

• Common Uses: Tinctures made from berries or fruit, such as elderberry or cranberry, are known for their immune-boosting, antioxidant, and urinary tract health benefits.

Whole Plant:

• Extraction Method: Some tinctures utilize the whole plant, including stems, leaves, flowers, and sometimes roots. This method captures a broad spectrum of active compounds.

• Common Uses: Tinctures made from the whole plant may offer a comprehensive range of benefits, combining various properties for overall wellness. Herbs like St. John's Wort or nettle might be used in this manner.

• Ensure the plant material is clean, free from contaminants, and properly identified.

• Adjust the extraction method and duration based on the specific plant part being used to extract the maximum medicinal properties.

• Follow appropriate ratios of herb to solvent for optimal extraction and potency.

• Store the tinctures properly in airtight, dark glass containers to preserve their potency.

Different plant parts yield diverse concentrations of active compounds, allowing for a wide spectrum of therapeutic applications in tincture making, catering to various health needs and preferences.

Choosing herbs for tincture making involves considering several factors to ensure efficacy, safety, and the desired therapeutic effects. Here's a step-by-step guide on how to select herbs for tincture preparation:

• Identify Health Needs: Understand the specific health concerns or goals you aim to address, whether it's immune support, stress relief, digestive health, etc.

• Study Herb Properties: Research the medicinal properties, uses, and contraindications of different herbs. Understand their active compounds and how they align with your intended purpose.

• Source High-Quality Herbs: Choose reputable suppliers offering organically grown or sustainably harvested herbs to ensure quality and potency. Confirm authenticity and avoid contaminants or adulteration.

• Select Suitable Plant Parts: Determine whether leaves, flowers, roots, bark, berries, or other parts of the plant are most suitable for addressing your health concerns based on their medicinal properties.

- Check Safety Profile: Consider any potential allergies, interactions with medications, or contraindications associated with specific herbs. Consult with an herbalist or healthcare professional if unsure.

- Preference and Tolerance: Consider personal preferences in taste, smell, and tolerance levels for certain herbs. Some may prefer or tolerate certain flavors or sensations better than others.

- Create Blends for Synergy: Some herbs work well together synergistically. Consider creating blends or combining herbs to enhance their effects or target multiple health issues simultaneously.

- Start with Small Batches: Begin with smaller batches when experimenting with new herbs or combinations to assess their efficacy and individual tolerance.

- Consider Harvest Time: Some herbs are more potent when harvested at specific times. Freshness can affect the quality of the tincture. Choose fresh or properly dried herbs for extraction.

• Ethical Considerations: Consider the sustainability and ethical harvesting practices of the herbs you select. Aim to support ethical and sustainable sourcing.

By considering these factors, you can choose herbs that align with your health goals, ensuring the creation of effective and safe tinctures. Always remember to research, seek guidance when needed, and start with small doses when trying new herbs to monitor their effects.

SAFETY CONSIDERATIONS WHEN CHOOSING HERBS FOR TINCTURE MAKING

When choosing herbs for tincture making, prioritizing safety is crucial to ensure the efficacy and well-being of individuals using the herbal preparations. Here are key safety considerations:

• Accurate Identification: Ensure accurate identification of herbs to prevent misidentification or use of toxic look-alike plants.

• Authenticity: Source herbs from reputable suppliers to avoid adulteration or contamination.

• Know Individual Allergies: Consider known allergies or sensitivities to specific herbs. Check for potential allergic reactions or cross-reactions with other substances.

• Consult with Healthcare Providers: Some herbs may interact with medications or have contraindications for certain health conditions. Consult healthcare professionals, especially if taking medications or having underlying health issues.

• Understand Toxicity Levels: Research potential toxicity levels of herbs. Some herbs, in high doses or prolonged use, may cause adverse effects.

• Proper Dosage: Adhere to recommended dosage guidelines. Start with smaller doses to assess individual tolerance.

• Safety during Pregnancy and Breastfeeding: Certain herbs are contraindicated during pregnancy or breastfeeding. Avoid herbs with potential adverse effects unless advised by a qualified healthcare provider.

• High-Quality Sources: Choose herbs from reputable sources to ensure they are free from contaminants, pesticides, or heavy metals.

• Ethical Considerations: Select herbs that are ethically and sustainably harvested to support conservation efforts and prevent over-harvesting of endangered species.

• Toxicity in Specific Parts: Some herbs have different toxicity levels in various parts (leaves, roots, seeds). Research and use appropriate parts safely.

• Gradual Introduction: When trying new herbs, introduce them gradually to monitor for any adverse reactions.

• Observation and Monitoring: Monitor for any unexpected reactions or side effects while using the tinctures.

• Avoid Unsafe Herbs: Avoid using herbs with a history of significant adverse effects or those without sufficient safety data.

Prioritizing safety considerations when selecting herbs for tincture making helps mitigate potential risks and ensures the safe and effective use of herbal preparations. When in doubt, seeking guidance from qualified herbalists or healthcare professionals is advisable, especially for individuals with underlying health conditions or those on medications.

THE MATERIALS NEEDED FOR HERBAL TINCTURES

To prepare herbal tinctures, several materials are required to ensure the proper extraction and storage of the tincture. Here's a list of materials along with their functions:

1. Herbs:

• Function: The primary ingredient, providing the medicinal properties and active compounds for the tincture.

• Consideration: Choose high-quality, properly identified, and dried or fresh herbs based on the desired medicinal effects.

2. Solvent (Alcohol, Glycerin, or Vinegar):

• Function: Acts as the extraction medium to draw out the active constituents from the herbs.

• Consideration: Select an appropriate solvent (e.g., high-proof alcohol like vodka or grain alcohol, glycerin for alcohol-free tinctures, or vinegar) based on the herb and desired tincture type.

3. Glass Jars or Bottles:

• Function: Used for maceration (soaking) of herbs in the solvent and for storing the prepared tincture.

• Consideration: Use clean, sterilized glass jars or bottles with tight-sealing lids to prevent contamination and preserve the tincture.

4. Labels and Markers:

• Function: Used for labeling jars or bottles to identify the herbs used, solvent type, preparation date, and any other relevant information.

• Consideration: Clearly label each tincture bottle to avoid confusion and ensure proper identification.

5. Strainer or Cheesecloth:

• Function: Used for straining the herbs from the solvent after maceration to separate the liquid extract from solid plant material.

• Consideration: Use a fine-mesh strainer or multiple layers of cheesecloth to effectively strain the tincture.

6. Funnel:

• Function: Assists in pouring the tincture into bottles without spillage or wastage.

• Consideration: Choose a clean funnel appropriate for the size of the bottle neck to facilitate easy transfer of the tincture.

7. Measuring Tools (Measuring Cups or Scales):

• Function: Used for accurate measurement of herbs and solvents to maintain proper ratios in tincture preparation.

• Consideration: Use calibrated measuring tools for precision in herb-to-solvent ratios.

8. Labels or Stickers:

• Function: Used to label jars or bottles during the steeping period to keep track of the date of preparation and any other important details.

• Consideration: Labels or stickers should be adhesive and waterproof to prevent smudging or fading.

9. Storage Containers:

• Function: Used for storing extra or bulk herbs before tincture preparation, ensuring they remain dry and protected.

• Consideration: Choose airtight containers to maintain herb freshness and potency.

10. Dark-colored Bottles:

• Function: Protects the tincture from light exposure, which can degrade its potency over time.

• Consideration: Use amber or dark-colored glass bottles to store the finished tincture, preserving its medicinal properties.

By utilizing these materials appropriately, herbal tincture-making can be done effectively while ensuring the quality and potency of the final product.

CHAPTER TWO

Preparing herbs for herbal tinctures involves several steps to optimize their extraction and potency. Here's a guide on how to prepare herbs for tincture-making:

1. Herb Selection:

• Choose high-quality, organic herbs that are free from contaminants and pesticides. Both dried and fresh herbs can be used for tincture-making.

2. Cleaning and Inspection:

• Dried Herbs: If using dried herbs, inspect them for any debris or impurities and remove any damaged parts.

• Fresh Herbs: For fresh herbs, gently rinse them with water to remove dirt or debris. Pat them dry with a clean cloth or paper towel.

3. Cutting or Grinding:

• Dried Herbs: If the herbs are in larger pieces, consider grinding or crushing them to increase the surface area for better extraction.

• Fresh Herbs: For fresh herbs, finely chop or bruise them slightly to release their natural oils and enhance extraction.

4. Maceration:

• Place the prepared herbs into a clean, dry glass jar for tincture preparation. Ensure the jar is large enough to accommodate both the herbs and the solvent (alcohol, glycerin, vinegar, etc.).

5. Herb-to-Solvent Ratio:

• Determine the appropriate herb-to-solvent ratio based on the desired strength and potency of the tincture. Ratios vary depending on the herb and the solvent used.

6. Solvent Selection:

• Choose the appropriate solvent for the tincture, such as alcohol (ethanol), glycerin, vinegar, or oil, based on the herb's properties and intended use.

7. Maceration Period:

• Pour the chosen solvent over the herbs in the jar, ensuring they are fully covered. Seal the jar tightly with a lid.

• Allow the herbs to steep in the solvent for several weeks in a cool, dark place, away from direct sunlight. The maceration period typically ranges from 4 to 6 weeks, but it can vary based on the herb and the solvent used.

8. Agitation:

• Gently shake or stir the jar every few days during the maceration period to agitate the mixture, aiding in the extraction process.

9. Straining:

• After the maceration period, strain the tincture using a fine mesh strainer or cheesecloth to separate the liquid extract from the solid plant material. Squeeze the herbs to extract as much liquid as possible.

10. Bottling and Storage:

• Transfer the strained tincture into dark-colored glass bottles for storage. Label each bottle with the herb name, solvent used, and preparation date.

• Store the bottles in a cool, dark place to maintain the tincture's potency and efficacy.

Additional Tips:

• Ensure all equipment used is clean and sterilized to prevent contamination.

• Adjust herb preparation methods based on specific herb characteristics and recommended tincture-making guidelines for optimal results.

By following these steps and guidelines, you can effectively prepare herbs for herbal tinctures, extracting their beneficial compounds and creating potent herbal extracts suitable for various health and wellness purposes.

Safety is paramount when working with alcohol and herbs, especially in the context of making herbal tinctures. Several key considerations underscore the importance of safety in this process:

• Alcohol as a Solvent: Alcohol, often used as a solvent in tincture making, is highly flammable. Working in a well-ventilated area and away from open flames or sources of heat is crucial to prevent fire hazards.

• Safety Precautions: Handle alcohol with caution, avoiding spills and ensuring proper storage in a cool, dry place away from children and pets. Always use appropriate personal protective equipment (PPE), such as gloves and goggles, when handling alcohol.

• Individual Reactions: Herbs can cause allergic reactions or sensitivities in some individuals. Understanding potential allergic responses and ensuring proper identification of herbs can prevent adverse reactions.

• Avoid Toxic Herbs: Some herbs can be toxic if used inappropriately or in high doses. Proper identification and knowledge of herbs to avoid toxic varieties are critical.

• Accurate Identification: Ensure accurate identification of herbs to prevent the use of poisonous or misidentified plants.

• Clear Labeling: Accurate and clear labeling of tinctures, including the herb used, solvent type, preparation date, and any precautions or contraindications, is essential for safety and identification purposes.

• Consultation with Experts: Seek guidance from herbalists, healthcare professionals, or reputable sources to understand potential contraindications, interactions, and proper dosage of herbs, especially when preparing tinctures for specific health conditions or if on medications.

• Proper Ratios: Maintaining accurate ratios of herbs to solvent is crucial to ensure the efficacy and safety of the tincture. Follow recommended guidelines and measurements for tincture preparation.

• Secure Storage: Store tinctures safely, preferably in dark-colored glass bottles, away from direct sunlight and in a location inaccessible to children or pets.

• Hygiene and Cleanliness: Maintain proper hygiene and cleanliness during tincture preparation to prevent contamination. Wash hands, sanitize equipment, and ensure cleanliness of the work area.

• Trial and Observation: When trying new tinctures or herbs, start with smaller doses and observe for any adverse reactions or side effects before regular use.

Maintaining safety protocols and precautions when working with alcohol and herbs not only ensures the quality and efficacy of herbal tinctures but also minimizes potential risks and promotes the overall well-being of individuals involved in the tincture-making process and those using the final product.

THE IMPORTANCE OF CHOOSING HIGH-QUALITY HERBS AND THEIR SOURCING

Selecting high-quality herbs and ensuring their proper sourcing is critical for several reasons, particularly when preparing herbal tinctures:

• Active Constituents: High-quality herbs contain optimal levels of active constituents (phytochemicals, essential oils, etc.) necessary for therapeutic effects. This ensures the tincture's efficacy in delivering intended health benefits.

• Absence of Contaminants: Quality sourcing ensures herbs free from pesticides, heavy metals, or other contaminants that might compromise safety or cause adverse health effects.

• Correct Identification: Proper sourcing from trusted suppliers reduces the risk of misidentification or substitution with incorrect or adulterated plant material. Authentic herbs ensure the desired medicinal properties are obtained.

• Conservation of Resources: Sourcing from ethical and sustainable practices supports the preservation of plant species, ecosystems, and biodiversity. It prevents over-harvesting and promotes responsible use of natural resources.

• Optimal Growing Conditions: Herbs sourced from reputable growers often come from well-maintained, nutrient-rich soil and ideal growing conditions. This can enhance the herb's medicinal properties.

• Reliable Sources: Reputable suppliers often conduct quality testing, ensuring herbs meet specific standards for potency, purity, and absence of contaminants.

• Prevention of Adulteration: Reliable sourcing minimizes the risk of adulteration or dilution of herbs with lower-quality or substitute plant material, ensuring the authenticity of the herb.

• Consistent Effects: Using consistently high-quality herbs from reliable sources ensures consistent results in tincture preparations, maintaining reliability and predictability in their effects.

• Building Trust: High-quality sourcing builds trust among herbalists, practitioners, and consumers, fostering confidence in the safety and effectiveness of herbal tinctures.

• Compliance with Standards: Sourcing herbs from reputable suppliers often ensures compliance with legal regulations and industry standards regarding herb cultivation, harvesting, and distribution.

Choosing high-quality herbs and sourcing them from reputable and ethical suppliers is fundamental in ensuring the safety, efficacy, and reliability of herbal tinctures. It supports the responsible use of medicinal plants, contributing to their conservation and promoting the overall well-being of individuals using these natural remedies.

THE STEP-BY-STEP PROCESS OF MAKING HERBAL TINCTURES

Here's a step-by-step guide on how to make herbal tinctures:

Materials Needed:

• Herbs of choice

• Alcohol (such as vodka, brandy, or grain alcohol)

• Glass jar with a tight-sealing lid

• Labels and marker

• Cheesecloth or fine mesh strainer

• Funnel

• Dark-colored glass bottles for storage

Step-by-Step Process:

1. Herb Selection:

• Choose high-quality dried or fresh herbs based on the desired medicinal properties and purpose of the tincture.

2. Herb Preparation:

• If using dried herbs, crush or grind them to increase surface area for better extraction. Fresh herbs can be chopped or lightly bruised.

3. Herb-to-Alcohol Ratio:

• Determine the herb-to-alcohol ratio based on the herb type and strength desired. A common ratio is around 1 part herb to 4 or 5 parts alcohol, but this can vary based on the herb's potency.

4. Maceration:

• Place the prepared herbs in a clean glass jar.

• Pour the alcohol over the herbs, making sure they are fully submerged. Leave some space at the top of the jar.

• Seal the jar tightly with a lid.

5. Steeping Period:

• Store the jar in a cool, dark place, away from direct sunlight.

• Allow the herbs to steep in the alcohol for several weeks to extract their medicinal properties. Steeping times can vary but generally range from 4 to 6 weeks. Shake the jar gently every few days to aid extraction.

6. Straining:

• After the steeping period, strain the tincture using a fine mesh strainer or several layers of cheesecloth.

• Place the strainer over a clean bowl or another jar and pour the tincture through it to separate the liquid extract from the solid plant material.

7. Bottling:

• Use a funnel to transfer the strained tincture into dark-colored glass bottles for storage.

• Seal the bottles tightly with caps or dropper lids.

8. Labeling and Storage:

• Label each bottle with the name of the herb used, type of alcohol, preparation date, and any other relevant information.

• Store the labeled bottles in a cool, dark place to preserve the tincture's potency.

Additional Tips:

• Ensure all equipment used is clean and sterilized to prevent contamination.

• Check regularly during the steeping period to ensure the herbs remain fully submerged in alcohol.

• Research specific herb characteristics and recommended tincture-making guidelines for best results.

Following these steps allows for the creation of homemade herbal tinctures, capturing the medicinal properties of herbs in an alcohol-based extract suitable for various health purposes. Adjustments to the process can be made based on individual preferences or specific herbal requirements.

THE VARIOUS EXTRACTION METHODS AND THEIR PROS AND CONS.

There are several extraction methods used to create herbal tinctures, each with its own set of advantages and limitations. Here are some common extraction methods along with their pros and cons:

Alcohol (Ethanol) Extraction:

Pros:

• Efficient Extraction: Alcohol is a potent solvent, extracting a wide range of compounds from herbs, including both water-soluble and fat-soluble constituents.

• Long Shelf Life: Alcohol acts as a natural preservative, extending the tincture's shelf life.

• Fast Extraction: Compared to some other methods, alcohol extraction often achieves rapid extraction of herbal properties.

• Versatile: Works well for a broad spectrum of herbs, allowing for comprehensive extraction of active constituents.

Cons:

• High Alcohol Content: Some individuals may prefer alcohol-free preparations due to personal preferences, taste, or health reasons.

• Evaporation of Alcohol: During the extraction process, alcohol can evaporate, affecting the final concentration and potency of the tincture.

• Potential for Denaturing Certain Compounds: Some delicate constituents might be altered or denatured by high-proof alcohol.

Glycerin Extraction (Glycerites):

Pros:

• Alcohol-Free Option: Suitable for those avoiding alcohol-based tinctures due to personal or health reasons.

• Sweet Flavor: Glycerin-based tinctures have a sweet taste, making them more palatable, especially for children.

• Preservative Properties: Glycerin acts as a preservative, albeit less potent than alcohol, extending shelf life.

Cons:

• Limited Extraction of Compounds: Glycerin has lower solvent power compared to alcohol, resulting in a less comprehensive extraction of herbal constituents.

• Shorter Shelf Life: Glycerin-based tinctures have a shorter shelf life compared to alcohol-based tinctures.

• Potential for Spoilage: Glycerin-based tinctures may be susceptible to bacterial growth if not stored properly.

Vinegar Extraction (Vinegar Tinctures):

Pros:

• Acidic Extraction: Vinegar extracts water-soluble constituents and minerals effectively from herbs.

• Alcohol-Free Option: Suitable for those preferring alcohol-free preparations.

• Lower Cost: Vinegar is generally less expensive than alcohol or glycerin.

• Taste and Smell: Vinegar-based tinctures may have a strong taste or odor, potentially affecting palatability.

• Limited Solubility: Vinegar may not extract fat-soluble compounds as efficiently as alcohol.

• Potential for Spoilage: Vinegar-based tinctures have a shorter shelf life compared to alcohol-based tinctures and are susceptible to bacterial growth if not properly stored.

Oil Extraction (Oil Infusions):

Pros:

• Fat-Soluble Extraction: Suitable for extracting lipid-soluble compounds from herbs.

• Topical Applications: Herbal oils are often used topically for massages, skincare, and external applications.

Cons:

• Limited Versatility: Oil extractions are not suitable for oral consumption and have limited applications compared to alcohol or glycerin-based tinctures.

• Longer Extraction Time: Oil infusions often require a longer period for extraction compared to alcohol or glycerin.

Water Extraction (Decoctions and Infusions):

Pros:

• Simple and Traditional: Water extraction methods are straightforward and have been used traditionally for brewing teas or decoctions.

• Safe for Oral Consumption: Suitable for creating herbal teas or infusions meant for oral consumption.

Cons:

• Limited Extraction of Compounds: Water is not efficient in extracting certain fat-soluble compounds, limiting its efficacy in extracting the full spectrum of herbal constituents.

• Shorter Shelf Life: Water-based preparations have a shorter shelf life and may be prone to spoilage compared to alcohol-based tinctures.

Considerations:

• Herb Selection: Different extraction methods may suit certain herbs better based on their constituents (water-soluble or fat-soluble).

• Purpose of Tincture: The intended use (oral consumption, topical application) can influence the choice of extraction method.

Each extraction method has its advantages and drawbacks, and the selection of the method often depends on the properties of the herb, desired constituents, and the intended use of the tincture.

HOW TO CARRY OUT THE VARIOUS METHODS OF EXTRACTION

Alcohol (ethanol) extraction is a commonly used method for preparing herbal tinctures. Here is a step-by-step guide on how to carry out alcohol extraction:

Materials Needed:

- Herbs of choice (dried or fresh)

- High-proof alcohol (such as vodka, brandy, or grain alcohol)

- Glass jar with a tight-sealing lid

- Labels and marker

- Cheesecloth or fine mesh strainer

- Funnel

- Dark-colored glass bottles for storage

Step-by-Step Process:

1. Herb Selection:

- Choose high-quality herbs based on the intended use and medicinal properties required.

2. Herb Preparation:

• If using dried herbs, crush or grind them to increase the surface area for better extraction. For fresh herbs, chop or lightly bruise them.

3. Herb-to-Alcohol Ratio:

• Determine the desired herb-to-alcohol ratio based on the herb's potency and the strength of the tincture desired. Common ratios range from 1:4 to 1:5 (1 part herb to 4 or 5 parts alcohol).

Glycerin-to-Herb Ratio:

• Determine the desired glycerin-to-herb ratio. Common ratios range from 1:2 to 1:3 (1 part herb to 2 or 3 parts glycerin).

Vinegar-to-Herb Ratio:

• Determine the desired vinegar-to-herb ratio. Common ratios range from 1:2 to 1:3 (1 part herb to 2 or 3 parts vinegar).

Oil-to-Herb Ratio:

• Determine the desired oil-to-herb ratio. A common ratio is usually around 1:4 or 1:5 (1 part herb to 4 or 5 parts oil).

4. Maceration:

• Place the prepared herbs into a clean glass jar.

• Pour the high-proof alcohol over the herbs, ensuring they are completely submerged. Leave some space at the top of the jar.

• Seal the jar tightly with a lid.

5. Steeping Period:

• Store the jar in a cool, dark place away from direct sunlight.

• Allow the herbs to steep in the alcohol for several weeks to extract their medicinal properties. The steeping time can vary but generally ranges from 4 to 6 weeks. Shake the jar gently every few days to aid extraction.

6. Straining:

• After the steeping period, strain the tincture using a fine mesh strainer or several layers of cheesecloth.

• Place the strainer over a clean bowl or another jar and pour the tincture through it to separate the liquid extract from the solid plant material.

7. Bottling:

• Use a funnel to transfer the strained tincture into dark-colored glass bottles for storage.

• Seal the bottles tightly with caps or dropper lids.

8. Labeling and Storage:

• Label each bottle with the name of the herb used, type of alcohol, preparation date, and any other relevant information.

• Store the labeled bottles in a cool, dark place to preserve the tincture's potency.

Additional Tips:

• Ensure all equipment used is clean and sterilized to prevent contamination.

• Check regularly during the steeping period to ensure the herbs remain fully submerged in alcohol.

• Research specific herb characteristics and recommended tincture-making guidelines for best results.

Following these steps allows for the creation of alcohol-based herbal tinctures, extracting the medicinal properties of herbs in an effective manner suitable for various health purposes. Adjustments to the process can be made based on individual preferences or specific herbal requirements.

HOW TO CARRY OUT WATER EXTRACTION

Water extraction involves using water as a solvent to extract water-soluble compounds from herbs. There are two primary methods: decoction and infusion.

Decoction Method:

Materials Needed:

• Herbs of choice (usually tougher plant parts like roots, barks, seeds)

• Water

• Pot

• Strainer

Steps:

• Herb Preparation: Use dried or fresh herbs. If using tougher plant parts like roots or barks, consider chopping or crushing them to increase surface area.

• Water-to-Herb Ratio: Calculate the water-to-herb ratio. Use approximately 1 tablespoon of herb per cup of water.

• Boiling: Place the herbs and water in a pot. Bring it to a boil.

• Simmering: Once boiling, reduce the heat and let it simmer for about 20-30 minutes, or longer for tougher plant parts.

• Straining: After simmering, remove the pot from heat and let the decoction cool. Strain the liquid using a fine mesh strainer or cheesecloth into a clean container, separating the liquid extract from the herb material.

• Storage: Store the decoction in a sealed container in the refrigerator for immediate use or freeze it in ice cube trays for future use.

Infusion Method:

Materials Needed:

• Herbs of choice (usually softer plant parts like leaves, flowers)

• Water

• Heat-resistant container (such as a teapot or heatproof pitcher)

• Strainer

Steps:

• Herb Preparation: Use dried or fresh herbs. If using softer plant parts like leaves or flowers, crush or chop them slightly to release their flavors.

• Water-to-Herb Ratio: Determine the water-to-herb ratio. Use approximately 1 teaspoon of herb per cup of water.

• Boiling Water: Bring water to a boil in a kettle or pot.

• Steeping: Place the herbs in a heat-resistant container. Pour the boiling water over the herbs. Cover the container and let it steep for about 5-15 minutes, depending on the herb and desired strength.

• Straining: After steeping, strain the liquid using a fine mesh strainer or cheesecloth into a clean container, separating the liquid extract from the herb material.

• Storage: Use the infusion immediately or store it in a sealed container in the refrigerator for short-term use.

Additional Tips:

• Decoctions are suitable for extracting compounds from tougher plant parts, while infusions are better for delicate parts like leaves and flowers.

• Ensure clean and sterilized equipment to prevent contamination.

• Adjust the herb-to-water ratio and steeping time based on personal preferences and specific herb characteristics for desired potency.

Water extraction methods are ideal for creating herbal teas or infusions meant for oral consumption, providing a gentle way to extract water-soluble compounds from herbs. Adjustments to the process can be made based on individual preferences or specific herbal requirements.

THE IMPORTANCE OF PROPER MEASUREMENTS AND SANITATION

Proper measurements and sanitation play vital roles in various fields, including scientific research, culinary arts, healthcare, manufacturing, and more. Their significance cannot be overstated due to several reasons:

Importance of Proper Measurements:

• Accuracy and Precision: Accurate measurements ensure the reliability and correctness of results in experiments, formulations, and processes.

• Consistency and Reproducibility: Consistent measurements allow for reproducibility of experiments or processes, crucial for scientific validation and quality control in industries.

• Quality Control and Assurance: In manufacturing and production, precise measurements are critical for maintaining product quality and meeting industry standards.

• Safety Considerations: Incorrect measurements can lead to hazardous situations in chemical or pharmaceutical industries, affecting safety.

• Resource Management: Proper measurements aid in efficient resource allocation and usage, minimizing waste and optimizing productivity.

• Customer Satisfaction: In culinary arts or product manufacturing, accurate measurements ensure consistent taste, quality, and satisfaction for customers.

Importance of Sanitation:

• Health and Hygiene: Sanitation is fundamental in preventing the spread of diseases, infections, and illnesses in healthcare facilities, homes, and public places.

• Food Safety: Sanitation practices in food handling, storage, and preparation prevent foodborne illnesses and ensure food safety.

• Quality Assurance: Maintaining cleanliness and sanitation standards in manufacturing and production processes is crucial for product quality and compliance with regulations.

• Prevention of Contamination: Sanitation practices prevent cross-contamination in laboratories, healthcare settings, and food industries, ensuring integrity and purity of samples or products.

• Environmental Impact: Proper sanitation helps prevent pollution and protects the environment by reducing the spread of harmful substances or pathogens.

• Public Perception and Reputation: Sanitation standards significantly impact public perception, reputation, and trust in various industries and institutions.

Proper measurements and sanitation are integral components across diverse domains, ensuring accuracy, safety, quality, and hygiene. Adhering to standardized measurement techniques and maintaining high sanitation standards is crucial for efficiency, safety, and public health across multiple sectors, ultimately contributing to better outcomes, productivity, and well-being.

HOW TO MEASURE THE APPROPRIATE AMOUNT FOR TINCTURE MAKING

To measure the appropriate amount for tincture making, you'll need to consider the herb-to-solvent ratio, which determines the strength and potency of your tincture. The ratio varies based on the herb being used and the desired concentration of the final tincture. Here's a general guideline to help measure the appropriate amount:

Herb-to-Solvent Ratio:

For Dried Herbs:

• A common ratio is around 1:4 or 1:5 (1 part dried herb to 4 or 5 parts solvent). For example:

• Use 100 grams of dried herb for 400-500 milliliters (ml) of solvent (e.g., alcohol, glycerin, vinegar).

For Fresh Herbs:

• The ratio for fresh herbs might slightly differ due to their moisture content.

• Usually, a higher ratio of herbs to solvent is recommended for fresh herbs, such as 1:2 or 1:3.

• Weigh or Measure the Herbs: Use a kitchen scale to measure the amount of dried herbs required based on the herb-to-solvent ratio. For example, if the ratio is 1:5 and you need 100 grams of dried herb, measure it accurately.

• Calculate the Solvent Quantity: Based on the chosen ratio, determine the amount of solvent needed. For instance, for a 1:5 ratio with 100 grams of dried herb, you'll need 400-500 ml of solvent.

• Use Proper Measuring Tools: Use graduated measuring cups or beakers to measure liquids like alcohol, glycerin, or vinegar accurately. A kitchen scale can help measure liquids in grams if precise measurements are required.

• Maintain Consistency: Ensure consistency in measurements to reproduce similar tincture strengths and effects in subsequent batches.

• Adjust Ratios Based on Herb Potency: Some herbs may require higher or lower ratios depending on their potency. Research specific herb guidelines for tincture-making to adjust ratios accordingly.

• When in doubt, it's safer to start with a lower ratio and adjust it in subsequent batches based on the tincture's effectiveness.

• Record your measurements and the ratios used for future reference or modifications.

Always follow recommended guidelines, consider the herb's potency, and maintain accurate measurements to achieve desired concentrations and potency in your herbal tinctures. Adjustments can be made based on personal preferences and the intended use of the tincture.

CHAPTER THREE

The choice of alcohol and its proof (alcohol content) is a crucial consideration when making herbal tinctures. Here's an explanation of the factors influencing the choice:

Factors Influencing Alcohol Choice:

• Solvent Power: Alcohol acts as a solvent, extracting various compounds from herbs. Higher alcohol content typically results in more efficient extraction.

• Preservation: Alcohol acts as a natural preservative, extending the tincture's shelf life by inhibiting microbial growth and degradation of active constituents.

• Evaporation Rate: Higher-proof alcohol evaporates more rapidly. During the extraction process and over time, alcohol content may diminish due to evaporation.

• Taste and Palatability: The alcohol used affects the taste of the tincture. Some people prefer milder-tasting alcohols, while others may prefer higher-proof alcohols for stronger extraction despite a stronger taste.

• 70-95% Alcohol (140-190 proof): Commonly used for tincture-making due to higher solvent power, efficient extraction, and better preservation qualities. Ethanol (ethyl alcohol) is frequently used in this range.

• Lower Proof Alcohol (40-50%): Some individuals prefer lower-proof alcohol for tinctures due to taste considerations or personal preference. Vodka, which is typically 40% alcohol by volume, is a common choice.

Considerations when Selecting Alcohol for Tinctures:

• Herb Compatibility: Some herbs may benefit from higher-proof alcohols for more effective extraction, while others might be better suited to lower-proof alcohols for milder flavors.

• Intended Use: Consider the purpose of the tincture. For some applications, like children's tinctures, lower-proof alcohol or glycerin might be preferred.

• Personal Preferences: Taste, potency, and individual tolerance to alcohol can influence the choice of alcohol proof in tinctures.

• Regulatory Considerations: Depending on local regulations or personal beliefs, some individuals may prefer alcohol-free alternatives or lower-alcohol tinctures.

Safety Note:

• When working with high-proof alcohol, ensure proper ventilation and take necessary precautions due to its flammability.

The choice of alcohol and its proof in tincture-making depends on factors such as extraction efficiency, preservation, taste preferences, and the intended use of the tincture. Experimentation, herb-specific considerations, and personal preferences often guide the selection of the most suitable alcohol for creating herbal tinctures.

ALTERNATIVES FOR THOSE THAT PREFER NON-ALCOHOLIC TINCTURES

For those who prefer non-alcoholic alternatives or wish to avoid alcohol-based tinctures due to personal, health, or other reasons, several alternatives can be used as solvents for making herbal extracts. Here are some options:

1. Glycerin-Based Tinctures (Glycerites):

• Glycerin: Vegetable glycerin is a popular alcohol-free solvent used to create herbal tinctures, known as glycerites. It's sweet-tasting and suitable for children or those avoiding alcohol.

• Process: Follow similar procedures to alcohol-based tincture making, substituting alcohol with glycerin. The extraction time may be longer compared to alcohol-based tinctures.

2. Vinegar-Based Tinctures:

• Apple Cider Vinegar: Organic, unpasteurized apple cider vinegar is often used as a solvent for herbal extracts.

• Process: Similar to alcohol-based tinctures but using vinegar as the solvent. Vinegar-based tinctures have a sour taste and are commonly used for culinary and medicinal purposes.

3. Water-Based Tinctures:

• Water or Infusions: Herbal teas or infusions made by steeping herbs in hot water can extract water-soluble compounds.

• Process: Make strong herbal teas or infusions, allowing them to steep for an extended period. Water-based extracts are not as concentrated as alcohol-based tinctures but are suitable for certain herbs and purposes.

4. Oil-Based Extracts:

• Carrier Oils: Oils like olive oil, coconut oil, or almond oil can be used to create herbal oil infusions.

• Process: Infuse herbs in oil over a period to extract fat-soluble compounds. Oil-based extracts are suitable for external applications like massage oils, salves, or skincare.

• Extraction Efficiency: Different solvents extract different constituents. Some compounds are better extracted in alcohol than in glycerin or vinegar, so potency might differ.

• Taste and Preservation: Glycerin and vinegar may alter the taste of the tincture compared to alcohol-based versions. Also, they might have different preservation qualities.

• Usage and Application: Consider the intended use of the tincture. While glycerin-based tinctures are suitable for children, water-based extracts might be less concentrated and have shorter shelf lives.

Experimentation and consideration of specific herb properties and intended uses are crucial when choosing non-alcoholic alternatives for tincture making. Each solvent has its advantages and limitations, so it's essential to choose the best option based on individual preferences and requirements.

Filling the jar when making herbal tinctures is a crucial step to ensure proper extraction and preparation. Here's a detailed process of how to fill the jar when making herbal tinctures:

1. Prepare the Herbs:

• Select high-quality herbs based on your recipe or intended tincture.

• Clean the herbs by removing any debris, dirt, or damaged parts.

• Cut, crush, or chop the herbs according to the tincture recipe. This helps increase surface area and aids in extraction.

2. Choose a Suitable Jar:

• Use a clean glass jar with a tight-sealing lid. Ensure the jar is sterilized or thoroughly washed and dried to prevent contamination.

3. Herb-to-Solvent Ratio:

• Calculate the appropriate herb-to-solvent ratio based on the recipe or desired potency. This determines the quantity of herbs and solvent (alcohol, glycerin, vinegar, etc.) needed.

4. Layering the Jar:

• Place the prepared herbs into the jar. If using multiple herbs, consider layering them according to the recipe or your preferences.

• Fill the jar loosely with herbs, leaving some space at the top to allow room for the solvent.

5. Pouring the Solvent:

• Pour the chosen solvent (alcohol, glycerin, vinegar, etc.) over the herbs in the jar until they are fully submerged.

• Ensure the herbs are completely covered by the solvent to facilitate proper extraction. Add more solvent if necessary to cover the herbs entirely.

6. Removing Air Bubbles:

• Gently tap the jar on a countertop to help release any trapped air bubbles. This ensures that the solvent penetrates evenly throughout the herbs.

7. Seal the Jar:

• Securely seal the jar with a tight-fitting lid. Ensure it's closed properly to prevent leakage and to maintain an airtight environment.

8. Labeling and Dating:

• Label the jar with the name of the herb, type of solvent used, the date of preparation, and any other relevant information. This helps in identifying the tincture and tracking its preparation date.

9. Storing the Jar:

• Store the sealed jar in a cool, dark place away from direct sunlight or heat sources. This allows the herbs to macerate and extract their beneficial properties over time.

Additional Tips:

• Shake the jar gently after sealing to distribute the solvent evenly among the herbs.

• Check the jar periodically during the maceration period and top it off with more solvent if needed to ensure the herbs remain fully submerged.

Following these steps ensures proper filling of the jar, creating an environment conducive to herbal extraction and the creation of a potent and effective tincture. Adjustments can be made based on specific tincture recipes or individual preferences.

THE PROCESS OF SEALING THE JAR

Sealing the jar properly when making herbal tinctures is essential to maintain a controlled environment for the maceration process and prevent contamination. Here's a detailed process for sealing the jar:

• Prepare the Tincture: After filling the jar with herbs and solvent according to your recipe or desired ratio, ensure the contents are at the desired level and properly submerged in the solvent.

• Clean the Jar Rim: Wipe the rim of the jar thoroughly using a clean, dry cloth or paper towel. Ensure there are no herb particles, moisture, or spills on the rim that could affect the seal.

• Lid Inspection: Inspect the jar lid or cap to ensure it's clean and free from any debris or residues. Check for any dents or damages that might compromise the seal.

• Secure the Lid: Place the lid on the jar rim, making sure it fits snugly and aligns properly. Tighten the lid firmly by hand to create a secure seal. Avoid overtightening, which might damage the lid or jar threads.

• For added security, especially if using alcohol-based tinctures: Place a small piece of wax paper or parchment paper over the jar opening before screwing on the lid. This can help prevent the alcohol from corroding the lid.

• Check for Leaks: After sealing the jar, gently tilt it and inspect for any leaks or signs of liquid seepage around the lid. Tighten the lid further if needed.

• Labeling and Dating: Label the jar with the necessary information, such as the name of the herb, type of solvent used, the preparation date, and any specific notes or instructions. Use a waterproof marker or label.

• Store Properly: Place the sealed and labeled jar in a suitable storage location. Ensure it's stored in a cool, dark place away from direct sunlight or heat sources.

• Periodic Checks: Check the jar periodically during the maceration period to ensure the lid remains securely tightened and there are no signs of leakage or contamination.

Additional Tips:

• Use glass jars with proper sealing lids specifically designed for preserving food or tinctures.

• Ensure the jar and lid are thoroughly cleaned and dried before use to prevent contamination.

By following these steps, you'll seal the jar effectively, maintaining a controlled environment for the tincture-making process and ensuring the preservation of the herbs and solvent for optimal extraction and potency.

Daily shaking or agitation of herbal tinctures during the maceration process is crucial for several reasons, significantly influencing the tincture's potency and effectiveness. Here's why daily shaking is important:

• Improved Solvent-Herb Contact: Shaking the tincture jar daily helps in increasing the contact between the solvent (alcohol, glycerin, vinegar) and the herbs. This agitation aids in better extraction of active compounds by continuously agitating the mixture.

• Optimal Compound Release: Continuous movement helps break down the cell walls of the herbs, facilitating the release of active constituents into the solvent.

• Even Distribution of Extracted Compounds: Shaking the tincture ensures that the extracted compounds are evenly distributed throughout the solvent. This helps prevent concentration variances within the tincture.

• Avoids Herb Settling: Herbs can settle at the bottom of the jar during the maceration period. Shaking the jar helps prevent this settling, ensuring that all herbs are consistently exposed to the solvent.

• Maximizes Extraction Over Time: Continuous agitation ensures a consistent extraction process throughout the maceration period, maximizing the tincture's extraction efficiency.

• Promotes Consistency: Daily shaking contributes to a more consistent and potent tincture by maintaining a steady extraction process, leading to a more reliable end product.

• Potential Reduction in Maceration Period: Adequate and consistent shaking may help expedite the extraction process, potentially reducing the required maceration time to achieve desired potency.

• Maintains Active Involvement: Daily shaking also offers a sense of active involvement in the tincture-making process, ensuring proper care and attention to detail.

• Shake the tincture jar gently, but thoroughly, ensuring proper mixing without causing spills or leaks.

• Perform the shaking routine consistently each day to maintain an optimal extraction process.

Daily shaking is crucial during the maceration process as it significantly impacts the extraction efficiency, consistency, and potency of herbal tinctures. Consistent agitation ensures proper extraction of active compounds from the herbs, contributing to a high-quality and effective tincture at the end of the maceration period.

THE STEEPING DURATION

The steeping duration, also known as the maceration period, varies based on the herbs used in herbal tincture preparation. It refers to the duration during which the herbs steep in the solvent (alcohol, glycerin, vinegar, etc.) to extract their active compounds. The optimal duration is influenced by the specific properties of each herb and the intended potency of the tincture.

• Herb Type and Characteristics: Different herbs contain various compounds that extract at different rates. Some herbs release their active constituents quickly, while others may require a longer steeping period.

• Potency Desired: The intended strength or potency of the tincture influences the maceration period. Longer steeping durations often lead to stronger tinctures.

• Solvent Used: The type of solvent (alcohol, glycerin, vinegar, etc.) affects the extraction rate. Alcohol tends to extract compounds more efficiently compared to other solvents.

General Guidelines for Steeping Durations:

• Common Steeping Period: The standard maceration period for herbal tinctures typically ranges from 4 to 6 weeks. This duration is a good starting point for many herbs and is often recommended in recipes or traditional practices.

• Herb-Specific Considerations: Some herbs may require shorter or longer maceration periods:

a. Quick-Extracting Herbs: Herbs like lavender, chamomile, or lemon balm may need a shorter steeping duration, around 2 to 4 weeks, due to their high volatility.

b. Slow-Extracting Herbs: Harder plant parts like roots, barks, or seeds might require a longer maceration period, sometimes up to 6 to 8 weeks, for optimal extraction of their constituents.

Observation and Adjustment:

• Periodic Checking: Regularly monitor the tincture during the maceration period. Assess the color, aroma, and taste occasionally to gauge the extraction progress.

• Taste Testing: Some herbalists suggest tasting the tincture periodically to determine its strength. If the tincture is potent enough, it can be strained even before the set duration.

Tailoring the Process:

• Flexibility in Duration: While general guidelines exist, adjusting steeping durations is common in herbal tincture making. Experienced herbalists often tailor the process based on individual herb characteristics, personal preferences, and desired outcomes.

The steeping duration for herbal tinctures varies based on herb characteristics, solvent used, and the intended potency. While standard guidelines exist, adjusting the maceration period allows for customization, ensuring the extraction of optimal compounds and achieving the desired strength and efficacy in the final tincture.

HOW TO STRAIN THE TINCTURE AND TRANSFER IT INTO SUITABLE STORAGE BOTTLES

Straining the tincture and transferring it into suitable storage bottles is a critical step in the tincture-making process. Here's a detailed guide on how to strain and bottle the tincture:

Straining the Tincture:

Gather Necessary Materials:

• Fine mesh strainer, cheesecloth, or muslin cloth

• Funnel

• Clean glass bottles or jars for storing the strained tincture

• Prepare Straining Equipment: Place the strainer or cheesecloth over a clean bowl or another jar large enough to contain the strained liquid. Ensure the straining material is securely in place.

• Strain the Tincture: Pour the contents of the tincture jar into the strainer or through the cheesecloth-lined funnel. This separates the liquid (tincture) from the solid herb material.

• Pressing the Herbs: Use a spoon or clean hands to press the herb material in the strainer or cheesecloth. Extract as much liquid as possible while ensuring minimal herb particles pass through.

• Repeat Straining (Optional): For clearer tinctures, perform a second strain using a finer mesh or a fresh layer of cheesecloth to remove finer particles.

Transferring the Tincture to Storage Bottles:

• Prepare Clean Bottles: Ensure the glass bottles or jars for storage are clean, sterilized, and completely dry. Dark-colored glass bottles (amber or cobalt blue) are recommended to protect the tincture from light exposure.

• Using a Funnel: Place a funnel over the mouth of the storage bottle to avoid spills while pouring the strained tincture.

• Pouring the Tincture: Carefully pour the strained tincture into the storage bottles through the funnel. Fill the bottles to a suitable level, leaving a small airspace at the top.

• Labeling the Bottles: Label each storage bottle with the tincture name, preparation date, type of solvent used, and any additional relevant information. Use waterproof labels or a waterproof marker.

• Sealing and Storing: Seal the bottles tightly with their lids or caps. Ensure they are closed properly to prevent leakage.

• Store the labeled bottles in a cool, dark place away from direct sunlight or heat sources to preserve the tincture's potency.

Additional Tips:

• Consider using dropper bottles for convenient and controlled dosing.

• If storing multiple batches, label and organize them for easy identification.

• Store excess tincture that doesn't fit in the bottles in a separate, airtight container in a cool, dark place for future use.

Following these steps ensures a clean and efficient process of straining the tincture and transferring it into suitable storage bottles, preserving its potency and efficacy for extended use.

HOW TO PROPERLY STORE HERBAL TINCTURES TO MAINTAIN THEIR POTENCY AND SHELF LIFE

Proper storage is crucial to maintain the potency, efficacy, and shelf life of herbal tinctures. Here's a guide on how to store herbal tinctures appropriately:

Ideal Storage Conditions:

• Cool and Dark Environment: Store tinctures in a cool, dark place away from direct sunlight and heat sources. Exposure to light and heat can degrade the tincture's potency by accelerating the breakdown of active compounds.

• Stable Temperature: Aim for a consistent and moderate temperature range. Fluctuations in temperature can affect the tincture's stability and potency. Avoid storing tinctures in areas prone to temperature variations.

• Airtight Containers: Use airtight glass bottles or jars for storing tinctures. Dark-colored glass (amber or cobalt blue) helps protect the tincture from light exposure.

• Avoid Moisture: Keep tinctures away from areas with high humidity or moisture, as moisture can cause spoilage or microbial growth, reducing the tincture's shelf life.

• Labeling and Organization: Label each storage bottle with the tincture name, preparation date, type of solvent used, and any specific instructions. Organize bottles to easily identify and access different tinctures.

Shelf Life Expectancy:

Shelf life varies depending on factors such as the type of herbs used, the solvent used, and storage conditions. Generally:

• Alcohol-based tinctures: Can have a shelf life of 3 to 5 years when stored properly.

• Glycerin or vinegar-based tinctures: Shelf life might be shorter, typically around 1 to 2 years.

• Avoid Contamination: Use clean droppers or pipettes when dispensing tinctures to prevent contamination. Avoid touching the dropper tip to avoid introducing bacteria.

• Shake Before Use: Before each use, gently shake the tincture bottle to ensure even distribution of the extracted compounds.

Additional Tips:

• If sedimentation occurs, especially in glycerin-based tinctures, it's normal. Shake well before use to redistribute the settled particles.

• Store tinctures in a location accessible for regular use but away from children or pets.

• If storing multiple tinctures, consider grouping them based on frequency of use or type of herbal preparation.

• Consider noting any changes in color, smell, or taste, as these can indicate potential degradation or spoilage.

Proper storage is crucial to maintain the potency, quality, and shelf life of herbal tinctures. By storing tinctures in a cool, dark, airtight environment and following best practices, you can extend their shelf life and ensure their effectiveness over time. Regularly monitor and assess tinctures for any changes, and discard if there are signs of spoilage or degradation.

FACTORS THAT CAN AFFECT THE SHELF LIFE OF TINCTURES

Several factors can significantly impact the shelf life and stability of herbal tinctures. Understanding these factors helps in preserving the tincture's potency and efficacy. Here are the key elements that can affect the shelf life of tinctures:

• Freshness and Quality: The quality of herbs used directly influences the tincture's shelf life. Fresh, high-quality herbs tend to yield more potent and longer-lasting tinctures compared to old or poor-quality herbs.

• Alcohol vs. Non-Alcohol Solvents: The type of solvent used (alcohol, glycerin, vinegar, oil, water) affects the shelf life. Alcohol-based tinctures generally have a longer shelf life due to their preservative properties compared to non-alcoholic solvents.

• Light Exposure: Exposure to light, especially sunlight, can degrade the active compounds in tinctures. Storing tinctures in dark-colored glass bottles in a dark environment helps maintain potency.

• Temperature Fluctuations: Extreme temperatures or frequent fluctuations can impact the stability of tinctures. Storing them in a cool, stable environment helps preserve potency.

• Humidity and Moisture: Excess moisture can lead to microbial growth or spoilage. Storing tinctures in a dry environment prevents degradation.

• Seal Integrity: Airtight glass containers or bottles help prevent air exposure, which can oxidize and degrade the tincture over time.

• Over-Extraction: Prolonged extraction periods might lead to over-extraction of certain compounds, potentially affecting the stability and taste of the tincture.

• Proper Ratios: Using appropriate herb-to-solvent ratios ensures optimal extraction without overwhelming the solvent. Imbalanced ratios might affect the tincture's stability.

• Sanitation: Contamination during preparation or handling can shorten shelf life. Always use clean equipment and proper hygiene practices when making and dispensing tinctures.

• Freshness: Tinctures made more recently typically have a longer shelf life compared to older tinctures. However, proper storage practices are essential even for freshly made tinctures.

• Herb Composition: Some herbs inherently have longer shelf lives due to their constituents, while others may degrade faster.

Maintaining the potency and stability of herbal tinctures relies on factors such as quality of herbs, storage conditions, choice of solvent, and proper preparation. By controlling these variables and storing tinctures in suitable conditions, their shelf life can be extended, ensuring they remain effective for a more extended period. Regular monitoring, labeling, and observation of any changes help determine if a tincture is still suitable for use.

Recognizing signs of spoilage in herbal tinctures is crucial to ensure their safety and efficacy. Here are common signs indicating that a tincture might have spoiled or degraded:

Visual Signs:

• Mold or Growth: Visible mold growth or any unusual particles floating in the tincture indicate contamination or spoilage. Discard the tincture if you notice any growth.

• Color Changes: A significant change in color, especially darkening or cloudiness, from the original color of the tincture might indicate degradation or spoilage.

Smell and Taste:

• Foul Odor: A rancid or foul smell that is significantly different from the herb's usual aroma could indicate spoilage or contamination.

• Off-Taste: Tinctures that have gone bad may have an unpleasant or sour taste, unlike the typical taste of the herb or the tincture when freshly made.

• Separation: Visible separation of layers or sedimentation at the bottom of the tincture bottle, especially if it's excessive or unusual, can indicate spoilage.

Other Observations:

• Cloudiness: Excessive cloudiness that doesn't dissipate after shaking might signal spoilage or improper extraction.

• Expired Shelf Life: If the tincture has passed its expected shelf life (as per general guidelines), it's essential to evaluate its appearance, smell, and taste for signs of degradation.

What to Do if You Suspect Spoilage:

If you notice any of these signs or have concerns about the tincture's quality:

• Do Not Use: Avoid using the tincture if you suspect spoilage or degradation.

• Discard Safely: Safely dispose of the tincture by pouring it down the sink with plenty of water or into the trash, sealed in a container to prevent accidental consumption or contact with pets.

• Follow proper storage guidelines: Store in a cool, dark place away from heat and light.

• Use airtight, clean glass bottles and avoid contamination during preparation and usage.

• Monitor tinctures periodically for any changes in appearance, smell, or taste.

Regular observation and using your senses to detect any unusual changes in appearance, smell, or taste are key to recognizing signs of spoilage in herbal tinctures. Promptly disposing of a spoiled tincture prevents potential health risks and ensures the use of safe and effective herbal preparations.

CHAPTER FOUR

Determining the appropriate dosage for different tinctures involves considering several factors, including the herb used, individual factors such as age and health condition, and the tincture's strength or potency. Here's a guideline on how to determine dosage:

General Dosage Considerations:

• Start Low and Gradually Increase: Begin with a lower dosage and gradually increase if needed. This helps gauge individual tolerance and effectiveness.

• Consult Reliable Sources: Refer to reputable herbalists, published literature, or reliable sources for dosage recommendations specific to the herb or tincture.

• Individual Factors: Consider individual factors such as age, weight, health condition, and sensitivity to herbs when determining dosage.

• Consult Herbal Resources: Refer to reputable sources, herbal books, or websites specializing in herbal medicine. They often provide recommended dosages for various tinctures.

• Follow General Guidelines: For many adults, a standard dosage range might be around 20-40 drops (approx. 1-2 mL) of tincture diluted in water or juice, taken 2-3 times per day. However, this can vary widely based on the herb and its intended use.

• Adjust for Potency: Adjust dosage based on the tincture's potency. Stronger tinctures might require lower dosages, while milder ones might need higher amounts.

• Consider Herb-Specific Dosages: Some herbs have specific dosage recommendations based on their potency, intended use (e.g., medicinal vs. nutritional), and potential side effects.

• Individual Response: Monitor individual responses to the tincture. Some people might require a lower or higher dosage based on their body's reaction and the desired effect.

• Chamomile: 30-60 drops (1.5-3 mL) diluted in water, up to 3 times per day for relaxation or digestive support.

• Echinacea: 30-40 drops (1.5-2 mL) diluted in water, 2-3 times daily for immune support during times of need.

• Valerian: 30-60 drops (1.5-3 mL) diluted in water before bedtime for sleep support.

• Ginger: 20-40 drops (1-2 mL) diluted in water, up to 3 times per day for digestive issues.

Safety Notes:

• Always follow recommended dosages and precautions specific to each herb.

• If uncertain or if dealing with a specific health condition, consult a qualified herbalist or healthcare professional for personalized guidance.

Determining the appropriate dosage for different tinctures involves careful consideration of various factors. Starting with general guidelines, adjusting based on potency and individual response, and seeking reliable sources for herb-specific dosages help ensure safe and effective use of herbal tinctures.

THE IMPORTANCE OF SEEKING GUIDANCE FROM AN HERBALIST OR HEALTHCARE PROFESSIONAL

Seeking guidance from an herbalist or healthcare professional is crucial when using herbal tinctures, as their expertise can significantly impact your safety, efficacy, and overall well-being. Here's why it's essential to seek their guidance:

1. Knowledge and Expertise:

• Herbalist's Expertise: Herbalists have in-depth knowledge of herbs, their properties, interactions, and appropriate dosages. They can provide tailored guidance based on individual needs.

• Healthcare Professional's Insight: Healthcare professionals, including doctors or pharmacists, can offer insights into potential interactions between herbal remedies and medications, ensuring safety and preventing adverse reactions.

2. Personalized Recommendations:

• Individualized Approach: Herbalists and healthcare professionals can assess your specific health concerns, medical history, allergies, and ongoing medications to recommend suitable herbal remedies or dosages tailored to your needs.

3. Safety and Risk Management:

• Avoiding Complications: They can advise on potential side effects, contraindications, and interactions between herbs and medications to prevent adverse effects or complications.

• Identification of Risks: Professionals can identify any pre-existing conditions or health risks that may contraindicate certain herbs or require specific precautions.

4. Monitoring and Follow-Up:

• Health Monitoring: Professionals can monitor your progress, assess the effectiveness of herbal treatments, and make necessary adjustments for optimal health outcomes.

5. Reliable Information:

• Access to Trusted Resources: They have access to reputable sources, evidence-based information, and clinical experience, ensuring accurate and reliable guidance on herbal remedies.

6. Education and Empowerment:

• Educational Opportunities: Herbalists and healthcare professionals offer education on herbal remedies, empowering individuals to make informed decisions about their health.

When to Seek Professional Guidance:

• When considering herbal remedies for specific health concerns or chronic conditions.

• If taking medications or undergoing medical treatments to avoid potential interactions.

• If experiencing adverse reactions or uncertainty about proper usage or dosages.

Seeking guidance from an herbalist or healthcare professional is vital for safe and effective use of herbal tinctures. Their expertise, personalized recommendations, risk management, and access to reliable information are invaluable in ensuring that herbal remedies complement your health regimen safely and effectively.

VARIOUS ADMINISTRATION METHODS

Herbal tinctures offer various administration methods, providing flexibility in their usage. Here are several common administration methods for herbal tinctures:

1. Oral Administration:

• Direct Ingestion: Adding the recommended dosage directly into the mouth and swallowing. This method allows for quick absorption into the bloodstream.

• Dilution in Water or Juice: Mixing the tincture drops in a small amount of water or juice to mask the taste and make it more palatable before consumption.

2. Sublingual Administration:

• Sublingual Absorption: Placing the tincture drops under the tongue and holding them there for a short duration before swallowing. This allows for quick absorption of the tincture's constituents directly into the bloodstream through the mucous membranes.

3. Topical Application:

• Skin Absorption: Applying tincture directly to the skin for absorption. This method is common for localized treatments, such as using arnica tincture for muscle soreness or calendula tincture for skin conditions.

4. Inhalation:

• Steam Inhalation: Adding a few drops of herbal tincture to hot water for steam inhalation. This method is beneficial for respiratory issues or congestion.

5. Gargling or Mouthwash:

• Gargling: Diluting the tincture in warm water for gargling to soothe throat conditions or promote oral health.

6. Adding to Food or Beverages:

• Culinary Use: Incorporating tinctures into cooking or beverages for flavoring or added medicinal benefits. For instance, adding ginger tincture to tea or using vanilla tincture in recipes.

7. Eye or Ear Drops (Specialized):

• Careful Application: In specialized cases and under professional guidance, highly diluted tinctures might be used as eye drops or ear drops for specific conditions.

Safety Precautions:

• Always follow recommended dosages.

• Consult an herbalist or healthcare professional for appropriate administration methods specific to your health concerns or conditions.

• Dilute tinctures properly when using them for sensitive areas like the eyes or ears.

Herbal tinctures offer multiple administration methods, allowing for versatility in their usage. The choice of administration method often depends on the type of herb, the intended use, and personal preferences. Understanding these methods enables individuals to utilize herbal tinctures effectively based on their specific needs and preferences.

Each administration method for herbal tinctures offers distinct benefits based on the intended use, convenience, and effectiveness. Here are the benefits associated with the various administration methods:

1. Oral Administration:

• Quick Absorption: Direct ingestion allows for rapid absorption of the tincture's active constituents into the bloodstream, facilitating faster effects.

• Convenience: Simple and straightforward method for most individuals, especially when mixed with water or juice to mask the taste.

2. Sublingual Administration:

• Rapid Absorption: Placing tincture drops under the tongue allows for direct absorption into the bloodstream, bypassing the digestive system and offering quick effects.

• Bioavailability: Sublingual absorption enhances bioavailability, ensuring a higher proportion of active compounds are absorbed.

3. Topical Application:

• Localized Effect: Direct application to the skin targets specific areas for localized relief from pain, inflammation, or skin conditions.

• Ease of Application: Simple application method, and tinctures can be easily blended into creams or lotions for topical use.

4. Inhalation:

• Respiratory Relief: Steam inhalation with tinctures can provide relief for respiratory issues like congestion, cough, or sinus problems.

• Direct Action: Inhalation allows the active compounds to reach the respiratory tract directly, offering faster relief.

5. Gargling or Mouthwash:

• Oral Health: Using tinctures for gargling helps in maintaining oral hygiene and alleviating minor throat discomfort.

• Antimicrobial Action: Some herbal tinctures used for gargling have antimicrobial properties that can support oral health.

6. Adding to Food or Beverages:

• Versatility: Incorporating tinctures into food or beverages offers a convenient and enjoyable way to consume herbs, imparting both flavor and medicinal benefits.

7. Eye or Ear Drops (Specialized):

• Precision Application: Highly diluted tinctures used as eye or ear drops under professional guidance offer localized relief for specific eye or ear conditions.

Safety Precautions:

• While these methods offer various benefits, it's crucial to use them safely and in accordance with recommended dosages and professional advice.

The diverse administration methods for herbal tinctures provide flexibility and cater to different needs. Selecting the appropriate method depends on the intended use, the desired speed of action, and personal preferences. Understanding the benefits of each method allows individuals to utilize herbal tinctures effectively for their specific health concerns or conditions.

FEW POPULAR HERBS FOR TINCTURES AND THEIR SPECIFIC USES AND DOSAGES

Here are a few popular herbs commonly used for tinctures, along with their specific uses and general dosage guidelines:

1. Echinacea (Echinacea purpurea):

Uses: Boosts the immune system, supports upper respiratory health, and assists in fighting infections like colds and flu.

Dosage:

• Adults: Around 30-40 drops (1.5-2 mL) of tincture diluted in water, 2-3 times per day.

• Children (under guidance): Lower doses according to age and weight.

2. Valerian (Valeriana officinalis):

Uses: Promotes relaxation, helps with anxiety, and aids in improving sleep quality.

Dosage:

• For Sleep: 30-60 drops (1.5-3 mL) of tincture before bedtime.

• For Anxiety: Smaller doses, around 20-30 drops (1-1.5 mL), 2-3 times daily.

3. Chamomile (Matricaria chamomilla):

Uses: Calms the nervous system, aids in digestion, and promotes relaxation.

Dosage:

• For Relaxation: 30-60 drops (1.5-3 mL) of tincture in water, up to 3 times per day.

• For Digestive Support: Similar dosage as for relaxation.

4. Milk Thistle (Silybum marianum):

Uses: Supports liver health, aids in liver detoxification, and offers antioxidant properties.

Dosage:

• Standard: 30-40 drops (1.5-2 mL) of tincture, 2-3 times per day.

• For Specific Liver Support: Follow practitioner recommendations for dosages based on individual needs.

5. St. John's Wort (Hypericum perforatum):

Uses: Helps with mild to moderate depression, supports mood, and offers mild sedative effects.

Dosage:

• For Depression: Around 30-40 drops (1.5-2 mL) of tincture, 2-3 times per day.

• Under Professional Guidance: Dosage may vary based on individual conditions and response.

6. Lemon Balm (Melissa officinalis):

Uses: Calms nerves, promotes relaxation, and supports cognitive function.

Dosage:

• For Relaxation: 30-40 drops (1.5-2 mL) of tincture in water, up to 3 times per day.

Important Notes:

• Dosages provided are general guidelines. Always start with lower doses and gradually increase if needed.

• Specific dosages can vary based on the tincture's strength, individual responses, age, weight, and health conditions.

• Always consult an herbalist or healthcare professional for personalized recommendations, especially when using herbs for specific health concerns or combining them with medications.

These popular herbs for tinctures offer diverse health benefits, and their dosages vary based on individual needs and intended uses. It's crucial to consider individual factors and seek professional guidance for appropriate dosing to ensure safe and effective use of herbal tinctures.

COMMON HEALTH ISSUES OR AILMENTS AND SUITABLE HERBAL TINCTURES FOR THEM

Here's a list of common health issues or ailments along with suggested herbal tinctures that are often used to address or alleviate these conditions:

1. Anxiety and Stress:

• Herbal Tinctures: Chamomile, Valerian, Passionflower, Lemon Balm, Skullcap.

2. Insomnia or Sleep Issues:

• Herbal Tinctures: Valerian, Passionflower, California Poppy, Chamomile, Hops.

3. Digestive Problems:

• Herbal Tinctures: Peppermint, Ginger, Chamomile, Fennel, Meadowsweet.

4. Immune Support:

• Herbal Tinctures: Echinacea, Elderberry, Astragalus, Andrographis.

5. Cold and Flu:

• Herbal Tinctures: Echinacea, Elderberry, Garlic, Andrographis, Oregano.

6. Respiratory Issues:

• Herbal Tinctures: Mullein, Thyme, Eucalyptus, Elecampane, Marshmallow root.

7. Pain and Inflammation:

• Herbal Tinctures: Arnica, Turmeric, Willow Bark, Devil's Claw, Ginger.

8. Skin Conditions:

• Herbal Tinctures: Calendula, Plantain, Comfrey, Chickweed, Burdock root.

9. Women's Health (Menstrual Issues):

• Herbal Tinctures: Black Cohosh, Chaste Tree (Vitex), Dong Quai, Raspberry leaf.

10. Men's Health (Prostate Health):

• Herbal Tinctures: Saw Palmetto, Pygeum, Nettle root, Pumpkin Seed.

Important Notes:

• These suggestions are not exhaustive and may vary based on individual responses, health conditions, and interactions with medications.

• Always consult an herbalist or healthcare professional for personalized recommendations, especially when addressing specific health concerns or combining herbs with medications.

Herbal tinctures offer a diverse range of remedies for various health issues. Selecting the appropriate tincture often depends on the specific health concern, individual responses, and the herb's known properties. Seeking professional guidance ensures safe and effective use of herbal tinctures for specific health ailments or conditions.

Here are dosage recommendations and necessary precautions or contraindications for herbal tinctures commonly used for various health issues:

1. Anxiety and Stress:

Herbal Tinctures: Chamomile, Valerian, Passionflower, Lemon Balm, Skullcap.

Dosage Recommendations:

• Chamomile: 30-60 drops (1.5-3 mL) in water, up to 3 times daily.

• Valerian: 30-60 drops (1.5-3 mL) before bedtime.

• Passionflower: 30-40 drops (1.5-2 mL) up to 3 times daily.

• Lemon Balm: 30-40 drops (1.5-2 mL) up to 3 times daily.

• Skullcap: 30-40 drops (1.5-2 mL) up to 3 times daily.

• Avoid combining sedative herbs if using medications that induce drowsiness.

• Use caution during pregnancy or breastfeeding.

• Consult a healthcare professional for prolonged use or with existing health conditions.

2. Insomnia or Sleep Issues:

Herbal Tinctures: Valerian, Passionflower, California Poppy, Chamomile, Hops.

Dosage Recommendations:

• Valerian: 30-60 drops (1.5-3 mL) before bedtime.

• Passionflower: 30-40 drops (1.5-2 mL) up to 3 times daily.

• California Poppy: 30-40 drops (1.5-2 mL) before bedtime.

• Chamomile: 30-60 drops (1.5-3 mL) in water, up to 3 times daily.

• Hops: 30-40 drops (1.5-2 mL) before bedtime.

• Avoid alcohol when using sedative herbs.

• Consult a healthcare professional before use, especially when combining with medications or during pregnancy.

Important Note:

• The dosages provided are general guidelines. Individual responses and appropriate dosages may vary. Always start with lower doses and gradually increase if needed.

3. Digestive Problems:

Peppermint (Mentha × piperita):

• Uses: Alleviates symptoms of indigestion, gas, and bloating.

• Dosage: Around 20-30 drops (1-1.5 mL) diluted in water, up to 3 times daily.

• Precautions: Avoid high doses as they might cause heartburn or irritation in some individuals.

Ginger (Zingiber officinale):

• Uses: Aids digestion, relieves nausea, and helps with upset stomach.

• Dosage: Similar to peppermint, around 20-30 drops (1-1.5 mL) in water, up to 3 times daily.

• Precautions: Use caution with high doses, especially in individuals with gallstones or those taking blood-thinning medications.

Chamomile (Matricaria chamomilla):

• Uses: Soothes the digestive tract, helps with indigestion and stomach discomfort.

• Dosage: Typically 30-60 drops (1.5-3 mL) in water, up to 3 times daily.

• Precautions: Avoid if allergic to ragweed, daisies, or related plants. Use caution before surgery or with anticoagulant medications.

Fennel (Foeniculum vulgare):

• Uses: Assists in relieving gas, bloating, and indigestion.

• Dosage: Start with lower doses, around 20-30 drops (1-1.5 mL), and adjust as needed.

• Precautions: Exercise caution if allergic to celery, carrots, or related plants.

Important Notes:

• Always start with lower doses and gradually increase if needed while monitoring for any adverse reactions.

• If you have any existing health conditions, are pregnant, nursing, or taking medications, consult with a healthcare professional before using herbal tinctures for digestive issues.

• Some herbs may have specific contraindications or interactions with medications, so individual considerations are crucial.

4. Cold and Flu:

Echinacea (Echinacea purpurea or Echinacea angustifolia):

• Uses: Supports immune function and may reduce the severity and duration of cold symptoms.

• Dosage: About 30-40 drops (1.5-2 mL) in water, 2-3 times daily during illness.

• Precautions: Avoid prolonged use, especially in individuals with autoimmune disorders or allergies to daisies, ragweed, or related plants.

Elderberry (Sambucus nigra):

• Uses: Helps reduce cold and flu symptoms, possesses antiviral properties.

• Dosage: Typically 30-40 drops (1.5-2 mL) in water, 3-4 times daily during illness.

• Precautions: Use caution with raw or unripe elderberries; they should be properly prepared before consumption.

Garlic (Allium sativum):

• Uses: Exhibits antimicrobial properties, supports immune function.

• Dosage: About 30-40 drops (1.5-2 mL) in water, up to 3 times daily during illness.

• Precautions: High doses may cause gastrointestinal discomfort; consult a healthcare professional if taking blood-thinning medications.

Oregano (Origanum vulgare):

• Uses: Possesses antiviral and antibacterial properties.

• Dosage: Typically 20-30 drops (1-1.5 mL) in water, up to 3 times daily during illness.

• Precautions: Highly concentrated; ensure proper dilution. Prolonged use can affect beneficial gut flora.

Important Notes:

• Always adhere to recommended dosages and monitor for any adverse reactions or interactions.

• If you have underlying health conditions, are pregnant, nursing, or taking medications, consult with a healthcare professional before using herbal tinctures for cold and flu.

5. Immune Support:

Echinacea (Echinacea purpurea or Echinacea angustifolia):

• Uses: Supports immune function and may reduce the severity and duration of illnesses.

• Dosage: About 30-40 drops (1.5-2 mL) in water, 2-3 times daily for immune support.

• Precautions: Avoid prolonged use; use caution in individuals with autoimmune disorders or allergies to daisies, ragweed, or related plants.

Astragalus (Astragalus membranaceus):

• Uses: Enhances immune function, may help prevent colds and respiratory infections.

• Dosage: Typically 30-40 drops (1.5-2 mL) in water, 2-3 times daily for immune support.

• Precautions: Long-term use may affect blood pressure or blood sugar levels; consult a healthcare professional if diabetic or taking blood pressure medications.

Elderberry (Sambucus nigra):

• Uses: Possesses antiviral properties, supports immune health.

• Dosage: Generally 30-40 drops (1.5-2 mL) in water, 2-3 times daily for immune support.

• Precautions: Use caution with raw or unripe elderberries; ensure proper preparation before consumption.

Reishi Mushroom (Ganoderma lucidum):

• Uses: Supports immune function, possesses adaptogenic properties.

• Dosage: About 30-40 drops (1.5-2 mL) in water, 2-3 times daily for immune support.

• Precautions: Can potentially interact with certain medications; consult a healthcare professional if taking medications.

Important Notes:

• Follow recommended dosages and consider individual responses.

• Consult a healthcare professional before using herbal tinctures for immune support, especially if pregnant, nursing, have underlying health conditions, or taking medications.

6. Pain and Inflammation:

Turmeric (Curcuma longa):

• Uses: Anti-inflammatory properties, aids in reducing pain and inflammation.

• Dosage: Typically 30-40 drops (1.5-2 mL) in water, 2-3 times daily for pain relief.

• Precautions: May interact with certain medications; consult a healthcare professional if on blood-thinning medications or have gallstones.

Arnica (Arnica montana):

• Uses: Helps relieve muscle soreness, bruising, and joint pain.

• Dosage: Applied topically in diluted form; avoid internal use due to toxicity concerns.

• Precautions: External use only; do not apply to broken skin or open wounds.

Devil's Claw (Harpagophytum procumbens):

• Uses: Eases joint pain and inflammation.

• Dosage: Generally 30-40 drops (1.5-2 mL) in water, 2-3 times daily for pain relief.

• Precautions: Avoid if allergic to aspirin or have peptic ulcers; consult a healthcare professional if on medications.

Ginger (Zingiber officinale):

• Uses: Exhibits anti-inflammatory properties, assists in pain relief.

• Dosage: Similar to turmeric, around 30-40 drops (1.5-2 mL) in water, 2-3 times daily.

• Precautions: Use caution with high doses, especially in individuals with gallstones or taking blood-thinning medications.

7. Skin Conditions:

Calendula (Calendula officinalis):

• Uses: Soothes irritated skin, aids in wound healing, and reduces inflammation.

• Dosage: Applied topically as a diluted solution; 10-15 drops (0.5-0.75 mL) in a carrier oil or water.

• Precautions: Generally safe for external use; avoid if allergic to plants in the Asteraceae family.

Chamomile (Matricaria chamomilla):

• Uses: Calms and soothes irritated skin, possesses anti-inflammatory properties.

• Dosage: Similar to calendula, used as a diluted solution for topical application.

• Precautions: Use caution if allergic to ragweed, daisies, or related plants.

Lavender (Lavandula angustifolia):

• Uses: Known for its calming and skin-soothing properties.

• Dosage: Applied topically; 10-15 drops (0.5-0.75 mL) diluted in a carrier oil or water.

• Precautions: Generally safe for topical use; some individuals may have skin sensitivities.

Plantain (Plantago major):

• Uses: Supports wound healing, soothes skin irritations, and possesses anti-inflammatory properties.

• Dosage: Applied topically as a diluted solution; similar to other herbal tinctures, 10-15 drops (0.5-0.75 mL).

• Precautions: Safe for external use; discontinue use if skin irritation occurs.

8. Menstrual Issues:

Dong Quai (Angelica sinensis):

• Uses: Supports menstrual health, may help regulate menstrual cycles and ease menstrual cramps.

• Dosage: Typically 30-40 drops (1.5-2 mL) in water, up to 3 times daily during menstruation.

• Precautions: Avoid during pregnancy; consult a healthcare professional if taking blood-thinning medications.

Chaste Tree (Vitex agnus-castus):

• Uses: Supports hormonal balance, may alleviate premenstrual symptoms and irregular cycles.

• Dosage: Generally 30-40 drops (1.5-2 mL) in water, 1-2 times daily during the menstrual cycle.

• Precautions: Avoid during pregnancy or while breastfeeding; consult a healthcare professional if on hormonal medications.

Black Cohosh (Actaea racemosa):

• Uses: Alleviates menstrual discomfort, including cramps and menopausal symptoms.

• Dosage: Typically 30-40 drops (1.5-2 mL) in water, up to 3 times daily during menstruation.

• Precautions: Avoid during pregnancy; use caution in individuals with liver disorders.

Red Raspberry Leaf (Rubus idaeus):

• Uses: Supports uterine health, may reduce heavy menstrual bleeding and cramping.

• Dosage: About 30-40 drops (1.5-2 mL) in water, 1-2 times daily during the menstrual cycle.

• Precautions: Generally considered safe, but consult a healthcare professional if pregnant or have underlying health conditions.

9. Prostate Health:

Saw Palmetto (Serenoa repens):

• Uses: Supports prostate health, may help alleviate symptoms of benign prostatic hyperplasia (BPH).

• Dosage: Typically 30-40 drops (1.5-2 mL) in water, 1-2 times daily.

• Precautions: Generally well-tolerated, but consult a healthcare professional if on medications or have existing medical conditions.

Pygeum (Prunus africana):

• Uses: Supports urinary function, potentially beneficial for prostate health.

• Dosage: About 30-40 drops (1.5-2 mL) in water, 1-2 times daily.

• Precautions: Avoid if allergic to almonds or related plants; consult a healthcare professional if on medications.

Nettle Root (Urtica dioica):

• Uses: Helps support urinary flow and overall prostate health.

• Dosage: Typically 30-40 drops (1.5-2 mL) in water, 1-2 times daily.

• Precautions: Generally safe; consult a healthcare professional if pregnant, nursing, or taking medications.

Pumpkin Seed (Cucurbita pepo):

• Uses: Supports urinary and prostate health.

• Dosage: Similar to other tinctures, around 30-40 drops (1.5-2 mL) in water, 1-2 times daily.

• Precautions: Generally safe; consult a healthcare professional if allergic to pumpkin seeds.

Important Notes:

• Always adhere to recommended dosages and monitor for any adverse reactions.

• If you have underlying health conditions, are taking medications, or have concerns about prostate health, consult with a healthcare professional before using herbal tinctures.

Dosage recommendations for herbal tinctures used for anxiety, stress, insomnia, and related issues vary. It's essential to follow recommended dosages, consider individual factors, and seek professional advice, especially when dealing with specific health concerns, existing medical conditions, or using medications concurrently. Consulting a healthcare professional or an herbalist ensures safe and effective use of herbal tinctures.

POTENTIAL SIDE EFFECTS AND CONTRAINDICATIONS ASSOCIATED WITH CERTAIN HERBS

While herbs offer numerous health benefits, some individuals may experience side effects or contraindications. Here are potential concerns associated with specific herbs commonly used in tinctures:

1. Echinacea:

• Side Effects: May cause allergic reactions in individuals sensitive to daisies, ragweed, or related plants.

• Contraindications: Not recommended for individuals with autoimmune disorders or those taking immunosuppressants.

2. Valerian:

• Side Effects: Possible drowsiness, headache, dizziness, or gastrointestinal discomfort in some individuals.

• Contraindications: Avoid use with alcohol, sedatives, or medications that affect the central nervous system.

3. Chamomile:

• Side Effects: Allergic reactions in individuals allergic to ragweed, daisies, or related plants.

• Contraindications: Avoid use before surgery or when taking anticoagulant medications due to potential interactions.

4. St. John's Wort:

• Side Effects: Photosensitivity, leading to skin reactions in some individuals exposed to sunlight.

• Contraindications: Interacts with various medications, including antidepressants, birth control pills, and blood thinners.

5. Ginger:

• Side Effects: Potential gastrointestinal upset or heartburn in high doses.

• Contraindications: Caution advised for individuals with gallstones or those taking blood-thinning medications.

6. Milk Thistle:

• Side Effects: Rarely, individuals may experience mild gastrointestinal upset.

• Contraindications: Avoid use in individuals allergic to ragweed or other plants in the Asteraceae family.

Important Note:

• Always consult a healthcare professional or qualified herbalist before using herbal tinctures, especially if pregnant, breastfeeding, taking medications, or dealing with specific health conditions.

• Monitor for any adverse reactions or interactions when introducing new herbs or tinctures into your regimen.

While herbs used in tinctures offer numerous health benefits, certain individuals may experience side effects, allergies, or interactions. Understanding potential risks associated with specific herbs allows individuals to use herbal tinctures safely and seek professional guidance when needed. A personalized approach and professional advice are essential to ensure the safe and effective use of herbal remedies.

THE POSSIBILITY OF ALLERGIC REACTIONS TO HERBS

Allergic reactions to herbs, although relatively uncommon, can occur in some individuals. These reactions can range from mild to severe and may manifest as skin irritation, respiratory issues, gastrointestinal discomfort, or even anaphylaxis in rare cases. Here's an overview of the possibility of allergic reactions to herbs:

Causes of Allergic Reactions to Herbs:

• Pollen Allergies: Some herbs belong to plant families that may trigger allergic reactions in individuals allergic to specific pollens. For instance, ragweed-sensitive individuals might react to chamomile or echinacea.

• Cross-Reactivity: People with certain pollen allergies might have cross-reactivity to herbs that belong to the same botanical family. For example, those allergic to birch pollen might react to herbs like fennel, parsley, or carrots.

• Contact Allergies: Direct contact with certain herbs, especially in their raw form or essential oils, can cause skin irritation or allergic dermatitis in sensitive individuals.

Common Herbs That May Trigger Allergic Reactions:

• Echinacea: May cause reactions in individuals allergic to ragweed, daisies, or other plants in the Asteraceae family.

• Chamomile: Potential for allergic reactions in those sensitive to ragweed, daisies, or related plants.

• Fennel, Coriander, Parsley: Individuals allergic to birch pollen might react due to cross-reactivity with these herbs.

Managing Allergic Reactions to Herbs:

• Patch Test: Perform a patch test by applying a small amount of diluted herb on the skin to check for reactions before using it extensively.

• Start with Low Doses: Begin with small doses of herbal preparations and gradually increase while monitoring for any adverse reactions.

• Consult Healthcare Providers: Seek advice from healthcare professionals or allergists if you suspect allergies or experience any symptoms after using herbs.

• Discontinue Use: If an allergic reaction occurs, discontinue use immediately and seek medical attention if symptoms worsen or include difficulty breathing or swelling.

Allergic reactions to herbs are possible but relatively rare. Individuals with known allergies, especially to pollen or specific plant families, should exercise caution when using herbal remedies. Patch tests, starting with low doses, and seeking professional guidance can help mitigate potential allergic reactions and ensure safe usage of herbal preparations.

CHAPTER FIVE

When considering herbal tinctures for children, it's essential to approach their use cautiously and with careful consideration for the child's age, weight, specific health condition, and potential safety concerns. Some herbs might not be suitable for children, while others may require adjusted dosages. Here are a few considerations and commonly used herbal tinctures for children:

Considerations for Herbal Tinctures for Children:

• Dosage: Children typically require lower dosages than adults. Dosage recommendations vary based on the child's age, weight, and the herb used.

• Herbs to Avoid: Certain herbs might not be suitable for children due to potential risks or lack of sufficient safety data. Always consult a pediatrician or qualified herbalist before administering herbal tinctures to children.

Commonly Used Herbal Tinctures for Children:

Chamomile (Matricaria chamomilla):

• Uses: Calming, helps with digestion, and promotes relaxation.

• Dosage: Start with a very low dose and gradually increase if needed. A few drops in water or juice as recommended by a healthcare professional.

Catnip (Nepeta cataria):

• Uses: Mild sedative, aids in digestion, and may help with fever or colic.

• Dosage: Typically given in very small doses under guidance.

Lemon Balm (Melissa officinalis):

• Uses: Calms nerves, helps with digestion, and has mild sedative properties.

• Dosage: A few drops in water or juice under professional guidance.

Fennel (Foeniculum vulgare):

• Uses: Aids in digestion, helps with colic or gas issues in infants.

• Dosage: Small amounts as advised by a healthcare provider.

Ginger (Zingiber officinale):

• Uses: Assists with nausea, upset stomach, or motion sickness.

• Dosage: Administer in minimal amounts according to professional advice.

Important Note:

• Always seek guidance from a pediatrician or qualified healthcare professional before administering herbal tinctures to children.

• Start with very low doses and monitor for any adverse reactions or changes in the child's condition.

The use of herbal tinctures in children requires utmost caution, individualized dosages, and professional guidance. Consultation with healthcare professionals or herbalists helps ensure the safe and appropriate use of herbal remedies for children's specific health concerns or conditions.

HERBAL TINCTURES FOR PREGNANT OR NURSING WOMEN

Pregnancy and breastfeeding are sensitive periods, and caution should be exercised when considering herbal tinctures. Some herbs might be contraindicated due to potential effects on the developing fetus or the nursing infant. Here are considerations and commonly used herbal tinctures for pregnant or nursing women:

Considerations for Herbal Tinctures During Pregnancy and Breastfeeding:

• Safety Concerns: Not all herbs are safe for use during pregnancy or breastfeeding due to potential risks to the developing fetus or nursing infant.

• Professional Guidance: Consult a healthcare provider or a qualified herbalist before using herbal tinctures during pregnancy or breastfeeding to ensure safety and appropriateness for the individual.

Commonly Used Herbal Tinctures for Pregnancy or Nursing:

Ginger (Zingiber officinale):

• Uses: Helps alleviate nausea or morning sickness during pregnancy.

• Dosage: Generally considered safe in moderate amounts, but professional advice is recommended.

Raspberry Leaf (Rubus idaeus):

• Uses: Often used in the third trimester to support uterine health and prepare for childbirth.

• Dosage: Start with lower doses and gradually increase under guidance.

Herbs to Approach with Caution or Avoid:

• Echinacea: Some sources advise against its use during pregnancy due to immune-stimulating properties.

• St. John's Wort: Generally avoided during pregnancy or breastfeeding due to potential effects on mood and hormonal balance.

• Always consult a healthcare professional or qualified herbalist before using herbal tinctures during pregnancy or breastfeeding.

• Ensure that the herbal tinctures used are safe and do not pose any risk to the developing fetus or the nursing infant.

Pregnant or nursing women should approach the use of herbal tinctures cautiously and seek guidance from healthcare professionals or herbalists. Careful consideration of the safety and appropriateness of herbal remedies ensures the well-being of both the mother and the developing fetus or nursing infant.

HERBAL TINCTURES FOR THOSE WITH UNDERLYING HEALTH CONDITIONS

Individuals with underlying health conditions should exercise caution when using herbal tinctures, as certain herbs may interact with medications or exacerbate specific health conditions. Consulting a healthcare professional or qualified herbalist is crucial to ensure the safety and appropriateness of herbal remedies. Here are some considerations and commonly used herbal tinctures for individuals with underlying health conditions:

Considerations for Herbal Tinctures in Individuals with Health Conditions:

• Interactions with Medications: Some herbs might interact with medications, affecting their efficacy or causing adverse reactions.

• Potential Exacerbation: Certain herbs may worsen specific health conditions, such as liver disease, autoimmune disorders, or bleeding disorders.

Commonly Used Herbal Tinctures with Caution:

Ginger (Zingiber officinale):

• Uses: Assists with nausea, upset stomach, or motion sickness.

• Caution: Individuals on blood-thinning medications or those with gallstones should use ginger with caution.

Milk Thistle (Silybum marianum):

• Uses: Supports liver health and detoxification.

• Caution: Individuals with certain liver conditions or allergies to the Asteraceae family should use it cautiously.

Herbs to Approach with Caution or Avoid:

• St. John's Wort: May interact with various medications, including antidepressants, birth control pills, and blood thinners.

• Echinacea: Individuals with autoimmune disorders or taking immunosuppressants should avoid it due to potential interactions.

Important Note:

• Individuals with underlying health conditions should always consult a healthcare professional or qualified herbalist before using herbal tinctures.

• Discussing potential interactions, contraindications, and appropriate dosages is essential to ensure safe and effective use of herbal remedies.

For individuals with underlying health conditions, using herbal tinctures requires careful consideration and professional guidance to prevent adverse reactions or interactions with medications. Consulting healthcare professionals or herbalists helps tailor herbal remedies to individual needs while ensuring safety and efficacy.

CONCLUSION

In conclusion, herbal tinctures represent a time-honored and versatile form of natural remedies that have been cherished for their medicinal properties across cultures and generations. These concentrated herbal extracts offer a convenient and potent way to harness the therapeutic benefits of various plants.

From their historical roots in traditional medicine to their integration into modern healthcare practices, herbal tinctures continue to play a significant role in promoting holistic wellness. Their diverse applications, ranging from supporting the immune system, easing discomfort, aiding digestion, to promoting relaxation, highlight their versatility in addressing a wide array of health concerns.

However, their usage demands thoughtful consideration, ensuring proper selection of herbs, precise preparation methods, and understanding individual needs to maximize their efficacy and safety. Seeking guidance from qualified professionals, including herbalists or healthcare providers, is paramount, particularly when considering specific populations such as children, pregnant or nursing individuals, or those with underlying health conditions.

The art of crafting and using herbal tinctures not only emphasizes the importance of respecting nature's remedies but also underscores the significance of a holistic approach to health and wellness. With prudence, knowledge, and proper guidance, herbal tinctures stand as valuable allies in fostering well-being, offering a natural pathway toward balance and vitality in our lives.

www.ingramcontent.com/pod-product-compliance
Lightning Source LLC
Chambersburg PA
CBHW070939260726
48661CB00003B/1044